Sea Salt's Hidden Powers

Seasalt's Hidden Powers

The Biological Action of All Ocean Minerals on the Body and the Mind

Jacques de Langre, Ph.D.

Happiness Press
Magalia, California

℗1992
Happiness Press
P.O. Box DD
Magalia, CA 95954

Printed in the U.S.A.
11½th Edition

Library of Congress Catalog Card Number: 91-91188
ISBN 0-916508-42-0

Contents

ONE
Definition of Sea Salt
1

TWO
The Earth's Most Complex Substance
10

THREE
Salt and the Industrial Revolution
13

FOUR
What Natural Sea Salt Provides
15

FIVE
New Light on Mineral Supplements
21

SIX
Tracking Down Refined Salt
25

SEVEN
Raw Food and Salt
29

EIGHT
Cooking with Natural Sea Salt
35

NINE
Iodine-laden Breezes and Iodized Salt
43

TEN
How Nature Makes Iodine
48

ELEVEN
Radiation Fallout Protection
50

TWELVE
Sex, Salt and Your Kidneys
53

THIRTEEN
Salt Phobia
57

FOURTEEN
The Roots of Human Wisdom
62

FIFTEEN
Alchemy and Salt
67

SIXTEEN
Beginnings
82

SEVENTEEN
Most Often Asked Questions
84

Bibliography
91

Index
95

Definition of Sea Salt

T HERE is a truly natural sea salt that is obtained from the evaporation of the sea, simply, without artificiality or refining. The wind and the sun *only* dry the ocean brine that is channelled from the pure ocean waters into pristine shallow clay ponds, edged with watergrass and green plants. The dazzling white and clean crystals are briskly stimulated by the salt farmer, then hand-gathered daily from the flowing live saltwater ponds.

The truly sweet taste of this salt does satisfy the real hunger for salt that is a part of our instinct. It compels us to include in our daily food the most complex mineral element of the planet. It is that ocean salt alone which possesses the power to restore wholeness to the human internal seas, our body fluids.

When harvested with dedication and care, the oceans give us a natural sea salt with the most exquisite taste and a mix of physiologically-vital minerals. Today, every common table salt is artificial and sadly pales beside the real sea salt. Out of the richest spectrum of 92 essential minerals found in the ocean, the industrial refined variety retains only two! Debased while table salt deserves all of its bad name and all the crimes as charged.

Yet the real sea salt is good and indispensable for life. Biology and medical research vainly attemps to return trace elements and macro-nutrients to our diet. Real ocean salt offers us all of them and is capable of spelling the difference between life and death, health and illness, social sanity and planetary panic.

Sea Salt's Hidden Powers validates the body and mind functions that are helped and maintained by the minerals found in salt. This book also traces and documents the remaining world sources of natural sea salt, rare but thriving. Crystallized only by the heat of the sun, in the most pristine, least-polluted wild areas of the planet, the Celtic method of making salt saves valuable resources while preserving the vital marshlands, their fauna and flora. These culinary salts have their seal of identity, like vintage wines. Their purity, cleanliness and method of salt farming are substantiated by independent university research, and certified organic by a group of professional inspectors from "Nature et Progrès", which is Europe's most serious and prestigious consumer advocate organization.

Beware of "Sea salt" Labels

On the labels of almost every packaged food, in supermarkets as well as health food stores, from frozen and canned vegetables to breads and meats, the name "sea salt" appears often. Reading this, we may feel safe and reassured, thinking that here at least, when it comes to the salt part of the ingredients, all is well.

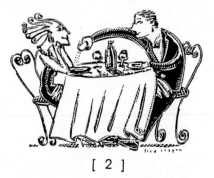

But All Is Not Well!

This sea salt has been totally refined. At its very origin, it may have come from the sea, but

1. it has been harvested mechanically from dirt and concrete basins with bulldozers and piped through rusted conduits;
2. subjected to many degrading artificial processes;
3. heated way beyond sun heat level in order to crack its molecular structure;
4. robbed of all of its essential minerals that are vital to our physiology;[1] and
5. further adulterated by chemical additives to make it free-flowing, bleached, and iodized.

To call what remains "sea salt" is a misnomer and a subterfuge.

In addition, harmful chemicals have been added to that vacuum processed, altered unnatural substance to mask and cover up all of the inequities it has suffered. These added chemicals include free flowing agents, inorganic iodine, plus dextrose and bleaching agents.

Where Do We Go from Here?

Both sides of the question have to be addressed. The simple, natural process of evaporation by sun power was scrapped[2] when consumers asked for a whiter-looking salt for the table and, later

---

1. These elements are extracted and sold separately to industry. Precious and highly prized by the salt refiners, these bring more profits than the salt itself.

2. In 1613, in Accomac County, Virginia, colonists from Great Britain dug shallow vats from rough-hewn trees and poured in sea water to let the sun dry the first sea salt. The news rang throughout the Virginia colony: "We will no longer depend upon England for our salt." Even if more significant than the 1773 Boston Tea Party, that kind of natural saltmaking in North America was short-lived, for in 1635 a patent was issued to Salem industrialist Samuel Winslow for a method of salt boiling and refining.

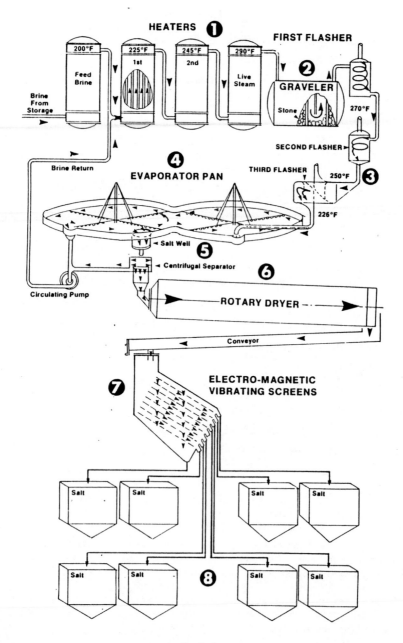

Part of the Process of Modern Salt Refining

Step 1: Brine enters a series of heaters which raise the temperature in several steps to 290° F. However, the brine does not boil at these high temperatures because it is kept under high pressure.

Step 2: Supercharged with heat, the brine enters the graveler, which is filled with cobblestones. Here the impurities are removed by being deposited like "boiler scale" because they are insoluble at such high temperatures.

Step 3: Next, the pressure is released in a series of flashers. This permits the brine to cool to 226° F and crystallization begins as the brine enters the last flasher.

Step 4: In the evaporator pan, salt crystals form, grow in size and are automatically raked into a large well. Brine not evaporated overflows at left and is pumped back to heaters for another trip through the process.

Step 5: The wet salt from the saltwell enters a centrifugal separator which removes most of the brine that is still in the salt. This brine returns to the heaters, while the salt goes to the rotary dryer.

Step 6: A continuous cascade of salt crystals passes down the rotary dryer through which a continuous blast of hot, filtered dry air is blown. This removes the remaining moisture and leaves the salt perfectly dry.

Step 7: Dried salt then flows over a series of magnetic screens ranging from 6 meshes per inch to nearly 100. Thus, salt for particular needs is precision screened.

Step 8: After screening and classification, each particular size of salt is stored in its own bin.

Diagram and captions courtesy of Diamond Crystal Salt Company, St. Clair, Michigan.

on, when industry demanded a chemically pure sodium chloride for the manufacturing of chlorine, plastic and for metallurgical and atomic energy uses. Profit-oriented salt makers discovered that huge benefits could be gained from the sale of several of these elements that are ripped off from the original sea brine. The mad greed race was on and the new industry of salt refining was born amid claims of purer, free-flowing whiter salt, half-truths and a barrage of propaganda. Salt had always represented integrity and truth; it is now another desecrated and scoffed-at fraudulent food substance.

Since human food salt consumption is only a mere seven percent of the total salt production — the balance, or 93%, is used by the chemical industry and manufacturing — very few people know that refined salt is a poison, and even fewer are aware that a whole and natural salt is still available. There is still one area of the world where true natural sea salt continues to be harvested whole and clean, proclaiming its integrity by a crystal form and its richness in minerals by its light gray coloring. It also possesses a label certifying its origin and organically-produced status, similar to the vintage wines of origin. Yet, refineries continue to vigorously promote their white shaker salt, all the while misleading consumers by calling it "sea salt."

Salt Farming, a Cottage Industry

Natural Celtic salt farmers proudly continue the age-old traditional salt making by the sea. Their single goal is to make a salt that enhances health and sharpens the mind. Only the sun and the wind are used for drying by these master saltcrafters as they harvest the crystals daily by hand and fastidiously maintain a clean, pristine environment around their salt farm.

The Celtic Brittany farmers continue to produce not only a salt that is friendly to human biology but one that also saves valuable forests and fuel, while preserving several thousand acres of vital pristine marshlands, its wild flora and fauna.

The micro-climate created by this vast network of forebays, channels, clearing reserve basins and evaporative shallow clay vessels contributes measurably to the region's healthful air and the planet's ecology. It also produces a natural salt that is the lowest in sodium and the richest in precious beneficial elements.

In August of 1991, the French government classified the salt-producing region of Brittany as a national shrine and recognized the practice of Celtic saltmaking as a national treasure.

Our ancestors long ago had recognized the life-giving and healing properties of sea salt. They also knew that natural crystal salt provided the vital connection with the forces and the elements of Nature. Therefore, it is worthwhile to spend a little time tracing the history of the extraction of salt in order to understand the vital role that this element has played in the development of human physical and mental welfare throughout history, as well as the great impact it continues to have in our spiritual life today.

Our forebears might have begun by using the rock salt of earth, the mineral element of the salt licks that animals used, or the salty brine from muddy water holes. Although rock salt deposits are not as desirable as natural sea salt, meat-eating nomadic tribes were able to adapt to higher concentrations of calcium sulfate and potassium chloride present in that earth salt because of their high meat diet. Vegetarians, however, do not fare as well on rock salt.

The red color of natural earth salt deposits together with a taste that resembles that of blood must have made a very profound impression on primitive tribes.

In the warmer climates, concentrating and drying the brine from salt springs and other sources was quite easy. After drawing buckets of salty water, many inland inhabitants ingeniously used hollowed tree trunks as vats to crystallize and de-bitter the salt. Most humans however had to wash then boil the salt brine in order to remove sand and dirt as well as excess potassium and calcium salts from it.

The more adventurous settlers camped near the seashore, becoming bolder and more independent in their thinking and in their deeds. Among these fearless early ancestors were the Celts, who recognized and held in high esteem three major symbols: wheat, water, and salt. These constitute a very strong trilogy of substances and a basis for their practical guiding principles of philosophy. Wheat is the symbol of life: the center, the regenerator of life. Salt is the extension of fire, issued from the waters, the powerful element used in alchemy and in transmutation. Crystal clear water and salt also bestow spiritual strength and virtuous morality.

Very deeply seated in the Celtic tradition is a reverence for the basic elements that surround the human race. Druidic priests performed seasonal rites of renewal on behalf of the tribe members. The forces of heaven and earth were known to meet and multiply in the cairn or rock cave. These were the wellspring of the priests' power as received from Nature.

The Druids, who were the Celtic people's secular leaders as well as their high priests, selected a wild and remote place — a mountain, an island, or a seashore — for their ceremonies, not only to avoid distraction but to be closer to nature's sacred forces. Curving loops of the great mystic spiral, carved inside the cairn, represent not only the journey of the soul moving through death to find rest and rebirth. Today, we still find that same spiral in a material, practical form as the very basic layout of the sunlit clay vessels/ponds carved near shores by the Celts for the extraction of salt from the ocean.

In making the seawater follow a spirallic course on land, the concentrated brine, about to be turned into moist crystals, retraces the same transmutation path that matter follows from chaos.

The Celts believed that sea salt, just like all natural elements, was endowed with special energetic properties and contained the spirit of the Deity. This has a logical verification in modern science, when one knows that sea salt is the product of earth's internal fire and the transmutation of tectonic rock layers by that fire under the bottom of the oceans. We also remember that the Celtic priests' function was to identify these forces of Nature and mark a clear path connecting those physical and spiritual elements to each member of the tribe.

Salt is the one element of transmutation in all of nature's substances that enables man to walk erect, gain intelligence, and remain totally free. This is why salt was so highly regarded and was actively gathered with great care every day. The cosmic origin of salt — which also connected us to our cradle of life, the ocean — was also known to have important significance. When salt is gathered from clay basins or from its micro-algae base, its ionization and strengthening is a result of a most intimate communion of salt and water with Heaven and Earth.

The careful scheduling and daily harvesting of the vital substance was, by tribal custom, always awarded to the most capable, positive and energetic men and women of the clan. Salt was the most precious element that was exchanged or given when meeting new people, a most enduring custom. Even now, when a gift is offered to another person, it is in the form of a small amount of genuine salt and a small loaf of wheaten or spelt bread. These remain the two traditional gifts of the Celtic people but many other cultures have adopted the practice.

┌─────┐
│ 2 │
└─────┘

The Earth's Most
Complex Substance

W HEN it is extracted from crystalline and clean windswept brine ponds, the ocean minerals in their entirety make the best quality food-grade salt. This fact was already recognized by the neolithic people, who had never studied natural biology or the physiology of salt, but intuitively understood that the salt from the sea was superior to that of land-locked salt licks. Instinct was their presentiment.

Throughout history, ocean salt has earned a hallowed reputation. Our ancestors saw it as an element that regenerates blood, a principle of equilibrium and life. To this day names of towns ending in "lick" still attest to the fact our that our early ancestors were drawn to the seashores or the rock salt deposits of the earth. In England town names ending in "wich," in Germany "saal," as in Salzburg, remind us of its neolithic origins. Early settlements grew up around these salt beds and springs.

The marked preference for sea salt over mine salt is deeply rooted in our genes. Today we still intuitively choose the product that states "sea salt" on the label, so strong is the age-old instinct. Today, however, that refined salt has the same identical chemical composition, whether it comes from the sea or from a land mine: it is 99% pure sodium chloride. All macro- and trace minerals are gone.

The commercial brands of today's table salt have not seen the sea for billions of years but comes from dried-up inland seas, dead salt lakes, or long-buried salt mines. Seventy percent of the salt produced today comes from fossil salt deposits.

There is no "natural sea salt" sold in any store. Even the bulk or packaged "sea salts" offered as natural in health food stores comes from the same refineries as the brand name salts. The macrobiotic-recommended salts such as Lima, Si-salt, Muramoto, etc. have been machine-harvested and either washed, boiled, skimmed and oven-dried. A comparison (overleaf) of their respective analyses, supplied by the makers or merchants themselves, tells much more than words.

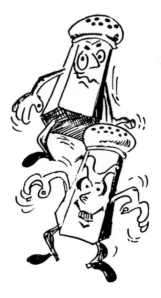

Comparison of the Mineral Elements in Natural Celtic Sea Salt vs. Other Salts

	Celtic Salt	Macrobiotic Salts	Refined Salt
Group 1			
Sodium & chlorine	84%	98%	97.5%
Group 2			
Sulfur, magnesium, calcium & potassium	14%	1%	none
Group 3			
Carbon, bromine, silicon,nitrogen, ammonium, fluorine, phosphorus, iodine, boron, lithium	1.9997%	1%	none
Group 4			
Argon, rubidium, copper, barium, helium, indium, molybdenum, nickel, arsenic, uranium, manganese, vanadium, aluminum, cobalt, antimony, silver, zinc, krypton, chromium, mercury, neon, cadmium, erbium, germanium, xenon, scandium, gallium, zirconium, lead, bismuth, niobium, gold, thulium, thallium, lanthanum, neodymium, thorium, cerium, cesium, terbium, ytterbium, yttrium, dysprosium, selenium, lutetium, hafnium, gadolinium, praseodymium, tin, beryllium, samarium, holmium, tantalum, europium	0.0003%	none	none
Group 5			
All chemical additives which bleach, prevent water absorption, stabilize iodine additives, maintain free flow	none	none	up to 2.5%

This analysis compiled by combining the research of University of Nantes, the work of Prof. L. C. Kervran, and the book by René Quinton, *Seawater: Organic Medium*, published by Library of the Medicine Academy, Paris, France.

$$\boxed{3}$$

Salt and the
Industrial Revolution

F ROM the mid-eighteenth century until World War I, the
economic history of salt making centers on a group of
changes known as the Industrial Revolution—the systematic
application of knowledge to the devising of more efficient production
methods. The science-based manufacturing of chemicals required
large quantities of salt (pure sodium chloride) for the industrial process
and factories. To save transportation costs, the industrial customers,
with their insatiable appetites for raw materials, located their plants
near salt works. From this new chemically-pure salt, they
manufactured explosives, chlorine gas, soda, agro-fertilizers and
plastics. These giant industrial complexes are also the salt makers'
biggest customers; they can spell which purity grade they wish as
well as influence which source will be exploited — namely, salt from
landlocked sources, which is already free of many minerals, already
dry, and therefore much cheaper to refine than ocean salt. Table
and food salt customers, being a rather insignificant part of the salt
market (7%), must bow to the decree of the industrial clients.

For the first time in the history of humanity, almost every country in the world now produces enough refined salt to insure its own industrial salt requirements at a most reasonable cost. However, if industrial-grade salt is cheap, when it comes to fulfilling the human biological needs, that modern wonder chemical is an expensive and dismal failure. If the effect of the Industrial Revolution has to be assessed in terms of human health, then we must look at the advent of the refining process as one of the major contributions to the breakdown of health in the modern world. Because refined salt is specifically formulated for industrial and chemical usage, there is little concern for the toxic effect of that salt on human biology.

Because table salt comes from the same batch as vacuum-refined industrial salt, it is treated with caustic soda or lime to remove all traces of magnesium salts. These vital magnesium salts are not taken out because they keep the salt from flowing out of the dispenser spout, it is because they bring in more profits on the chemical market. Yet these magnesium salts are a very necessary part of the food salt and fill important biological and therapeutic roles. Further, to prevent any moisture from being reabsorbed, salt refiners now add alumino-silicate of sodium or yellow prussiate of soda as desiccants plus different bleaches to the final salt formula. But since table salt, chemically treated in this way, will no longer combine with human body fluids, it invariably causes severe problems of edema (water retention) and several other health disturbances.

The fear of salt that we witness today and the virtual ban on consuming products with a high sodium content is a matter of serious concern to biologists. Salt-free diets can cause salt starvation, which is a stark reality of our modern world, but it is actually a starvation of macro- and trace minerals, a biological deficiency that refined sodium chloride alone cannot correct.

$$\boxed{4}$$

What Natural
Sea Salt Provides

T HE minerals that are present in sea salt, when ecologically extracted with manual dexterity and respect for life's laws, are the 84 elements that are originally in the sea. None of these elements are removed from natural Celtic sea salt. Once redissolved in water or in the moisture of food as it cooks, this re-created "ocean" bears an amazing likeness to human blood and body fluids. Basic physiology validates the fact that the ideal replenishing substance, capable of maintaining or restoring health in humans, would have to be that very sea salt that has retained all of the elements of original sea water. Although the biological necessity has not yet been proven for each of these elements, it has been established that 24 of these elements are essential to maintain life.[1] Many of these need only be present in parts per million (ppm) concentration in order to provide or restore essential biological functions. In fact, these

---

1. See *Scientific American*, July 1972: "The Chemical Elements of Life," by Earl Frieden.

trace elements are properly absorbed and utilized safely only when they occur in parts per million concentration. Here, concentration of these elements in excess of micro doses would cause clumping and provoke malabsorption in the living cells.[1]

Ocean minerals and dissolved gases, besides providing a stable environment for marine life, also help to maintain the chemical and physical stability of the living organisms based on dry land, assuring the survival of the planet's flora and fauna.

The air above the ocean waters becomes saturate with, distributes and constantly moves and releases the ocean's dissolved gases to all forms of land-based life around the globe. A large part of these airborne gases are destroyed by city pollution; luckily these same rare gases are locked within salt crystals as they form at the seashore, adding to the salt's effectiveness as biological regulators of our body's functions. Thus a clean and natural salt, with all these essential minerals and gases trapped within, is essential for effectively maintaining and restoring human energy. Interestingly, whenever natural Celtic sea salt is ground (not required or suggested) while being milled, the salt releases a subtle fragrance reminiscent of violets, another telltale sign that gases, floral-like vital essences, are being released.[2]

The Attributes of True Salt

Salt is such an important part of our food that very close scrutiny, attention and sensitivity must be given to the process used to produce

---

1. In his work on toxicology, Georges K. Davis (University of Florida) states: "A greater concentration increases the risk that these elements will form too strong an aggregation or clumping between them and therefore will no longer be free to make beneficial connections."

2. These elements are easily trapped and stored in a preparation called sesame salt. See recipe on page 35.

it so that the end product accurately fills our biological requirements. Most modern consumers are familiar only with the refined or boiled white, vacuum-evaporated product. To determine that a salt is a truly whole product of natural crystallization of the ocean, these guideposts will help. Only natural sea salt will have the following characteristics:

1. It is light gray in color and, on standing, the color darkens slightly at the base of the container.
2. It is moist to the touch and retains its moisture even when kept in cool storage for long periods.
3. It is formed of very small, precisely cubic crystals.

Each of these three signs proclaims the natural sea salt's integrity and wholeness but also guarantees its effectiveness as an outstanding food/condiment/medicine combination that builds, maintains or restores optimum health.

The Importance of the Gray Color

Some of the minerals present in true natural sea salt are responsible for the salt's light gray coloring and attest to its power to support all biological functions. Natural products reveal their richness in minerals by their color. It is true of whole wheat flour and natural unrefined sugar. By its total lack of color, white refined salt reveals its mineral deficiency and biological ineffectiveness.

Salt Moisture as a Vital Sign

The oceans are the lifeblood of the planet. All of the salt's essential trace and macro-elements stay within the crystal only as long as the moisture of that salt is retained. Applying any artificial heat will destroy the riches of the ocean while removing that moisture. If flash crystallized, kiln dried or boiled, the salt loses all. This water-retaining part of sea salt, centered around the magnesium salts that are highly water retentive, is called the mother liquor or bitterns. In the ancient traditional sacred medicine of the Celts, it is used to treat major physical and mental disturbances, severe burns, and other ailments. Today's biologists attest that the mother liquor restores hydro-electro-lytic imbalance, a disorder that causes the loss of immune response, creates allergies, and causes many health problems. The therapeutic effect of mother liquor is recognized and used by the European medical profession, and is still in use today. Moisture assists the transfer of the energy of the great oceans themselves; if the oceans are the lifeblood of our planet, then natural sea salt creates the lifeblood of our organism.

The moisture always present in Celtic natural salt settles at the bottom of the container or bag, leaving the top part almost dry to the touch. Thus it is always advisable to mix the contents of the salt bag before its use. Natural sea salt is best dispensed from a salt cellar or a salt box; it readily dissolves in the moisture of the food and is usually added near the end of the cooking. To sprinkle dry on food from a shaker makes the salt slightly harder to assimilate. In this latter form, it also enters the system in a non-ionized form, thus it can create thirst and lessen some of its advantages.

The Crystalline Structure and Its Quality

The small cubic crystals of natural sea salt hold and defend the integrity of this natural element. By presenting the least surface possible, water and oxygen cannot cross the cubic envelope and alter its contents. The cube shape forms an effective package for protection against outside influences. However, as soon as these crystals are broken or recrystallized, the salt's surface increases manifold and invites rapid oxidation and dehydration. At the same time, the faster and unrestricted evaporation of moisture out of the crystal dissipates a portion of the mother liquor, causing an even more pronounced loss of elements. Thus, this last sign, the sparkling crystal structure, has even more importance than the color, and proclaims the natural salt's integrity just as the brilliance of a gemstone affirms its worth.

These three signs of whole natural salt tell almost the entire story. The several thousand acres of salt marshes that produce Celtic ocean salt play a vital role of climatic regulators as well as thermic generators and accumulators. Every August (and we were able to witness this phenomenon during August of 1991) when the salt fields are ""cooking"" under the influence of superheated dry air, each sea storm front divides into two masses that lead any potential rain precipitation inland where they follow two distinct routes, one half of the front follows the Vilaine river while the other half follows the Loire valley. This reduces the rainfall below that of the Mediterranean sea. Additionally, the sunlit luminosity is that of high mountain regions, augmented further by the reflection of this light by the salt basins and the ocean.

To these climatic advantages, one must add an exceptional atmospheric quality since the off-land ocean winds, already charged with marine ions, further enriching themselves in oxygen, ozone, additional ions, and rare elements. Combined with the moisture evaporating from the salt flats, the combination forms huge ionized aerosol masses, totally free from land or urban pollution.

This marine ionized atmosphere bounces off the thick pine forests near these shores, where more vegetal quality oxygen is released to the salt crystals as they form. Further, since 1988, a quality control policy was adopted by the salt farmers, each harvest is selected for its uniformity of crystal. Such a selection is aimed at favoring and valorizing each small-scale harvest of an irreproachable quality based on a systematic determination of the quality of water and salt. Sifting the crystals eliminates any foreign bodies that might have been brought by the wind. This quality control has been officially distinguished by the Ministry of Agriculture that awarded the prestigious "Red Label," which is a hallmark of high-grade quality food product. In August of 1991, another acknowledgment by the prestigious Certified Organic Growers and Producers, "Nature et Progrès" of France, has given their recognition to the excellence of the salt field professionals.

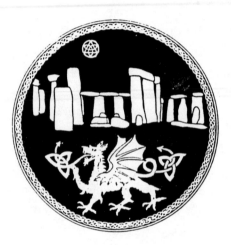

5

New Light on
Mineral Supplements

T is in the plant world that the major source of minerals for human nutrition is found: cereal grains, vegetables and fruits. Ocean salt, unrefined, entirely completes the requirements for essential elements, supplying trace minerals that are virtually unavailable from the plant world but are offered in "precise dosages" by the salt crystals. The controversy about taking dietary supplementation is still raging, especially if these are taken in inorganic form rather than through the vegetable realm. However, macro-nutrients as well as trace elements should never be taken carelessly in any quantity. Most of them have a very narrow quantitative range between what is essential and what is toxic. It is not enough, for instance, to have the proper quantity of the needed nutrients in one's diet; there is still the requirement that these trace elements be active and capable of being metabolized. Recent research[1] has shown that many of the physiological reactions of an organism are blocked and cannot

---

1. See Michel Deville's "Le Vrai Problème des Oligo-Éléments," *Centre de Recherches et d'Applications sur les Oligo-Éléments.* Bursins, France, 1978. Available only in French, it covers the "True Problem of the Trace Elements."

utilize trace elements properly. This malfunction can lead to simple deficiencies or to the initial establishment of illnesses.

Basic biology tells us that the activity of trace elements is most prominent at the level of enzymes that facilitate or regulate the organism's processes. Trace elements are seen as regulators, tending to harmonize the metabolic exchanges that assure normal reaction and function. Their presence endows an organism with the ability of self-restoration of its biochemical equilibrium. Without these trace elements, these processes would either be very slow or require excessive additional energy.

Of course, these reactions and functions occur only when very specific conditions are met as follows:

1. The right pH (acid/alkaline) of the ambient medium is maintained.
2. The rH_2 (oxydo-reduction potential) of the medium is achieved.
3. The temperature of the environment is correct.
4. The concentration, and correct relative percentage, of all elements exists.
5. The exact sequence of all prior reactions is followed (synergy of actions and reactions).
6. The rhythm follows the orderly cycle of life.
7. The other elements are present in their proper concentration (coactivity factor).

If a blocking of the organism occurs, it is possible to reactivate the enzymes by restoring the metallic salts—trace elements. But it has to be done in the form of an ionized solution of the metallic catalyzer in extremely low concentrations, as small as a few parts per million.

The need for the lowest possible concentration has been confirmed by the toxicology research of George K. Davis, at the University of Florida, which showed that metallic trace elements arrive more rapidly at the toxic dosage when they are ionized and therefore more readily assimilable.

Limiting the concentration of trace elements to less than parts per million is seen therefore as an imperative; it follows all of the recent recommendations of oligotherapy[1] and we sum up these findings below:

1. The supplementation of trace elements must be furnished in ionized form.
2. It must be administered in concentrations of parts per million or even less.

To illustrate the above point, let us compare ionized trace elements to the minute spark that serves to rekindle the "interest" of the organism for the already present but unused trace elements that lie dormant in the organism. In a blocked state, nothing happens until this "lightning" strikes.

Further, for a reaction to take place, it is necessary that the added particles achieve a bonded contact. In a solid state this is difficult to realize, but dissolved in liquids such as body fluids, the molecules are in motion and the shock that occurs within the solution readily storms up a chemical reaction. When any substance is dissolved in water, each molecule of the previously compact mass separates from the other, thus acquiring a mobility that allows it to roam about in the solute. The higher the temperature of the solution, the higher the velocity of its elements.

But often overlooked is the fact that too great a concentration of trace elements in an organism increases the risk of forming strong

---

1. A relatively new facet of biological medicine, oligotherapy is related to microchemistry and shows that a number of illnesses can be healed by the presence and action of metallic ions in the body: magnesium, iodine, iron and sodium at the infinitesimal molecular scale. The link between atoms plus the quantum mechanism of molecular orbits also enters into this science.

aggregations—clumping—of similar elements that cannot easily be freed from the solid mass, in order to serve as truly useful linkages with others on the outside.

The two points 1 and 2 cited on the previous page are the primary conditions that will assure a readily available supply of trace elements to an organism. Only when these two conditions are met will they be immediately mobile and thus usable. Unlike organic structures that must first be broken down in order to function, ionized trace element solutions immediately place all their elements instantly at the ready for transporting enzymes so that they instantly go wherever they are needed. Thus, the power of Celtic ocean salt lies in its infinitely small macro-nutrients: Boron, lithium, iodine, phosphorus, ammonium, strontium, and fluorine that make up 1.9997% of natural sea salt; as well as its trace elements: (See Group 4 on page 12): The fifty-four additional elements that occur only in micro-quantities. These account for only 0.0003% of natural gray sea salt; thus, each figures in parts per billion or even parts per trillion concentration.

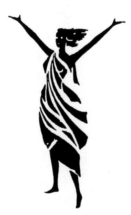

6

Tracking Down
Refined Salt

R EFINED salt is often labeled sea salt in supermarkets and natural sea salt in health food stores. Without any training, anyone can easily judge if a salt is truly unrefined and natural or if it is a fraud. To recognize a genuine sea salt, one need only look for these three signs:

1. A salt is natural and unrefined if the structure of each grain is made up of fairly small (3/16th of an inch) and very regular cubic crystals. Some refined salts, however, are recrystallized in large white crystals for certain markets such as road deicing, water softeners, cattle feed and kosher salt that only has to appear "natural" but is not.

2. Natural salt has a slight gray color, not white. However, the overall appearance of each crystal is one of clear sparkling brightness or luster. Some large crystal refined salts are often coated with glucose or other chemical to prevent them from sticking together and to allow them to pour easily. Most often, these crystals will then be of a dull, milky white appearance.

3. Pinching below the surface of the salt package, reach for a few grains, if the individual crystals feel damp and are moist enough to cling to the fingers, this is a "sun-dried only" ocean salt that has been stored properly after the harvest. Keeping in a cool and dark place helps to retain the protective moisture content and the precious mother liquor, which is the heart of the salt.

The Taste Test

Using the taste buds to track down refined salt is often the ultimate and most telling way. To establish the benchmark for the comparison, one or two crystals of Celtic salt are placed on the tongue and the saliva allowed to dissolve them. This is the guiding mark and once the flavor has been duly noted, the mouth is rinsed with clear water. A similar amount of the questioned salt is then tasted in the same way. This test is usually more than sufficient to decide if a new salt is genuine natural sea salt or a refined product that has been masquerading as the real thing.

The Lab Test

Should a more scientific test be required, one not based on personal taste, a test made in a laboratory of the University of California by biologist Jacques Loeb[1] can be duplicated with very little equipment by following the pioneering procedure. It will track down a refined salt without complex analysis. Dr. Loeb demonstrated that a pure sodium chloride (refined sea salt) solution, at the concentration in which the salt exists in sea water, is poisonous to marine organisms.

---

1. Jacques Loeb, M.D. and biologist, 1859–1924. During his years of professorship in the Biology Department of the University of California, besides his extensive study of the physiology of salt, he showed that fertilization was controlled chemically and separate from the transmission of hereditary traits.

The poisonous action of the sodium chloride was not due to the absence of the other constituents of sea water; young fish lived indefinitely in distilled water. It would, as Loeb remarks, be impossible to prove the toxicity of sodium chloride, if the organism were not able to live in distilled water. If Dr. Loeb's fish died in a solution of refined salt, what is the fate of our internal organs when fed commercial sodium chloride?

When the moisture inherently present in sea salt is forcibly removed by boiling, kiln-drying, or vacuum flash re-crystallization, the first essential elements to dissipate are magnesium salts. All other vitally important trace elements follow the leader and also leave whenever salt is mangled.

In refineries, salt is subjected to excessive heat, exhausting oxidation, and one or more bleaching agents are also used. Thus white refined salt is now bone-dry and sterile: it cannot maintain life. The salt makers' commercial advertisements state with pride that their product is 99.0% pure. This whiteness, however, is far from being a sign of excellence, it benefits only the chemical industry that buys 93% of the refineries' output. For such important customers, one can make concessions that hurt only a few other customers. The moisture present in natural sea salt assures us that it still contains the numerous elements that buffers the sodium chloride part of the salt and make up as much as 16% by weight in valuable trace elements and macro-minerals. Yet the Codex[1] standards for food salt states

---

1. The Codex or Codex Alimentarius is a collection of international food standards determined by a branch of the United Nations. It specifies standards for all major foods and with provisions for contaminants, food additives and analysis. As soon as the major industrialized nations accept a particular standard, it is incorporated in the world Codex and laws. The USDA Codex judged salt for its suitability for human consumption. Most processed foods have a Codex standard; vacuum refined salt is no exception. When the U.S. Codex asked the salt refiners for advice when drafting standards for table salt, the refiners obliged: sea salt must be 99% pure. "Impurities" include trace elements and macro-nutrients!

that sea salt shall not contain more than 2% of trace and extra minerals, other than sodium chloride. The salt sold in health food stores, even that which is labelled "sea salt," must conform to the same regulations and comes from the same refinery that produces toxic industrialized salt. Such sea salts as Lima, Si-salt and others have been purged of their minerals down to the 2% of macro-nutrients spelled out in the U.S. Codex.

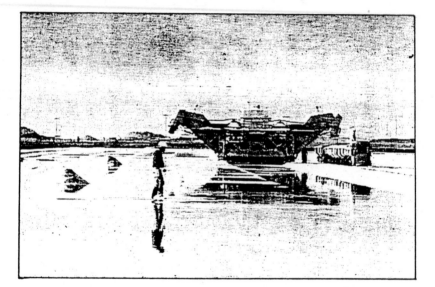

Raw Food
and Salt

THE earth gives forth an abundance of minerals that are best absorbed by humans in the form of vegetables, grains, and fruits. Moreover, the entire vegetal realm provides vitamins and enzymes from their living cells. Such an abundance of available nutrients has given some of us to the idea that vegetables alone, raw or cooked, could supply enough salt for one's diet. However, this is far from being the case.

In the wild, vegetarian animals consume large amounts of plants and grasses from their surroundings, and yet their constant grazing throughout the day cannot keep them supplied with enough salt to maintain their metabolism. Unless these beasts have access to earth salt licks or commercial salt blocks, the concentration of sodium chloride in all wild plants is so slight that many animal species invariably show marked evidence of sodium deficiency.

These same herbivorous animals do quite well without sodium chloride if nitrate deposits are accessible. Failing that, their constant grazing and nonstop chewing of wild vegetation never extract enough sodium or trace elements to satisfy their needs.[1]

On the other hand, domesticated, captive herbivorous animals—cows, sheep, horses, etc.—are fed cultivated grains and hay (not wild) that contain even less of these transmutable elements, and particularly NO magnesium salts. Herbivorous farm animals have to depend on salt blocks, the refined commercial kind of salt to which several chemicals have been added, such as antibiotics to prevent foot rot, insecticides to eliminate pesky flies and for other specific purposes such as putting on weight fast. These farm animals become acclimatized to and even become addicted to the chemically-altered salts just as humans have.

An even lower level of sodium chloride exists in cultivated vegetables and fruits, so that humans who rely solely on unsalted vegetarian fare are required to munch all day long on substantial amounts of greens and drink gallons of juice to make up for the lack of sodium that is a must for metabolic function.

In actuality, because fruits and vegetables are near salt-free, such a raw vegetarian diet will create an anemic condition and other salt-starvation diseases. This often triggers strong cravings for salted snack foods, or for rare meat as fresh killed animals --that have retained some urine and blood-- are not there to provide the needed salt.

A case in point is a well-known author of several books who advocates vegetarianism but no salt as well. She was often observed backstage eating rare steaks right after lecturing on the merits of vegetarian raw foods on the speaker's platform.

---

1. The salt licks they use contain more potassium nitrate than sodium chloride, and these animals are able to transmute at low energy. They make sodium chloride from potassium nitrate. According to Prof. Kervran in *Biological Transmutations* (see Bibliography), the formula is as follows: $K_{39} - O_{16} = Na_{23}$.

Another valid reason for adding salt to raw or cooked vegetable quality food is that the nutritive tissues of every plant are made up of complex carbohydrates; this constitutes one of the important food groups for humans and animals. Salt is the single element required for the proper breakdown of plant carbohydrates into usable and assimilable human food. Only when salt is added to fruits and vegetables can saliva and gastric secretions readily break down the fibrous store of carbohydrates. Thus here, as well as in cooked foods, an unsalted raw diet will not work.

Mine Salt is Meant for Meat Eaters

Certain aboriginal tribes who consume mostly fresh-killed animals have the life-preserving instinct of drinking the blood of their prey and also of cracking open the bones, sucking out the marrow and gnawing on the cartilages. Such steps increase the ratio of minerals to proteins. Such a step safeguards the heart and the health of these carnivorous humans.

Civilized peoples regularly consume aged meat that has had its blood drained out. Modern consumers never chew on the bones and cartilages of any beast. The proteins that they ingest are not neutralized by the minerals of the animal's marrow and blood. Such salt-poor proteins need to have minerals added, when they are absent, it causes a craving for extra salt. If a fresh kill could be consumed, this would provide the additional sodium, calcium and phosphorus needed for balance, but that is an instinct that has been lost by the meat-eaters of our modern civilization.

On such a blood-less meat diet, only no amount of salt reduction can check high blood pressure stemming from such an excessively high nitrogenous intake. We remember that both animal meat cause at least as much constriction as salt.

Why Mix Earth with Salt?

Today, the natives in some Pacific Islands, whose main diet is pork, still follow an inborn intuition of mixing a red ocher earth with the salt they sun-dry and harvest by hand from the sea. The earth veins are rich in iron and potassium nitrate, combined with their sea salt, this red alae earth supplies the missing elements that salt needs in order to balance their high fat and animal protein intake.

The instinct of these natives, whose consumption of meat requires more than just sodium chloride to keep in balance, biologically and automatically make or transmute what their body requires from added potassium salts. Previously, we saw that potassium-rich earth licks provided the missing element to carnivorous animals through a transmutation of potassium into sodium salts. The intuition that leads such meat eaters to seek and consume that special earth salt. The fact that it is totally safe to indulged in is yet another proof that biochemical and biological cravings are directed by faultless instinct.

Fertile Soil and Salt Minerals

Depleted soils and their reduced fertility cause a massive loss of trace minerals, as evidenced by analyses of the vegetation that grows on them. Market vegetables, called freeway crops, at best supply a mere fraction of the trace minerals essential for the proper function of the human body. Whole natural gray sea salt is fully mineralized and supplies a substantial part of the trace elements missing from today's overworked crops. Refined or white boiled salt, just like polished white rice, will not maintain life adequately. For nervous impulses to occur in an organism, there must be a difference of potential between the exterior and the inner part of its cells.

Even in the most primitive of cells, this is accomplished by an accumulation of potassium and magnesium inside the cell and a keeping of sodium and of calcium outside the cell. Only then is a gradient of concentration of sodium and potassium achieved. This creates a difference of potential between the outside and the inside of the cell. In the fluid that constantly bathes the cell, sodium is abundant. By maintaining osmotic pressure, that element effectively prevents excess loss of liquid. On the other hand, potassium, being the principal cation of the fluid inside the cell, serves to maintain the acid/alkaline balance of the inner medium.

In order to maintain these percentages of concentration of electrolytes on either side of the cell wall and to prevent losses of ions through its membrane, the cell spends a considerable part of its energy. Whenever a dietary deficiency of trace elements occurs, the cell loses its ability to control its ions — with dire consequences for humans. Even a minute loss of ion equilibrium causes cells to burst, nervous disorders, brain damage, or muscle spasms, as well as a breakdown of the cell regenerating process and growth.

This is why it is so vital that the saline and ionic composition of human blood be maintained within very precise limits. In other words, the concentration of sodium, potassium, magnesium and calcium must be kept constant and in proper relation to each other (coaction). If these relationships vary more than 1% above or below established limits, very noticeable pathological states occur.

An active transport of ions is insured across cell membranes by "pumps." These work to increase the internal concentration of potassium and also of magnesium + +. These same pumps also serve to lower the internal concentration of sodium + and of Calcium + +. According to the theory of acid and alkaline, chronic disease is caused by the acidification of the blood and the cellular tissues. This condition can be accurately measured by the pH of the patient's blood. The scale that is used for measuring the pH, or hydrogen ion concentration, runs from 0 to 14, with 7 being the neutral point, the pH of distilled water. The pH of a healthy person's blood is 7.35, whereas in a sick person the blood measures 7.30. Although this is only .05 more acid, this condition invites trouble, since this slight acid increase allows tissues and organs to easily become inflamed. The condition of acid blood, called acidosis, leads to various infectious diseases, liver illness, and aging problems such as neuralgia, rheumatism, cerebral hemorrhages, gastric ulcers and hypertension. Acidosis is very prevalent today. Unless this excess acidity is corrected by using a whole salt in the diet, acid-relieving medication do not work.

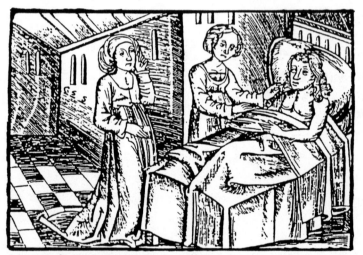

In earlier times, correcting the salinity of the internal body fluids ranked high in traditional medical practice. Many curative preparations then were elaborated from salt. Herbal teas, when lightly salted, propel the healing properties of the plant to the cell core.

8

Cooking with
Natural Sea Salt

N ATURAL sea salt in small crystal form dissolves easily for cooking, pickling, or baking. An additional benefit is that vegetables and cereal grains cooked with salt contain the electrolytes so vital to the life process. The chloride ions in natural seawater make up about 55% of its solids. Chlorine's function is to cleanse the toxins from the body and to combine with and move the sodium along to fulfill its many essential duties. Thus it is important to retain all the chlorine naturally occurring in sea salt. Boiling, kiln-drying, or pan-roasting removes a substantial part of the chloride, but it also destroys many of the other essential elements. For maximum health benefits, the salt should be added in its raw original crystal form to the food as it cooks, the moisture in the food rapidly dissolves it. Only in this manner will the salt and its other active co-nutrients be transmuted into regenerative blood cells along with the very elements of the food.

A delicious condiment which is also considered a very potent healing substance and a complement to any protein is sesame salt or "Gomashio." It can be easily be made as follows:

To prepare:
   1 cup unhulled sesame seeds
   1 level Tablespoon of Celtic sea salt

The traditional way to make sesame salt is to first rinse well in salt water,[1] rinse, drain, and lightly roast the sesame seeds until a nutty fragrance is reached and the seeds crush easily between thumb and ring finger. Quickly pour them out of the skillet. While the skillet is still hot[2] but with the flame turned off, the measured amount (usually one twelfth of the seed quantity) of salt is stirred until just dry. (Crush the salt first, or use the fine ground Celtic.) Combine both ingredients and grind together with mortar and pestle. As the roasted sesame seeds and the salt are ground together, the oil from the sesame seeds coats the salt crystals, making it easy for the body to assimilate. Salt consumed in its undissolved or uncooked form could cause thirst; in order to prevent this, salt should be added only during the cooking, and not sprinkled dry on the food at the table. In the form of this sesame salt however, it will not cause thirst. For fresh, raw fruits and vegetables: lightly sprinkled fine-ground Celtic, will greatly enhance their flavor while making these food more digestible.

When and Why to Salt Vegetable Foods

Salting vegetable foods is a necessity; the benefits of a vegetable

---

1. This step is necessary to remove the tannic and nicotinic acids from the outer bran coats of the sesame seeds. This step will remove the harsh, bitter taste from the seeds.

2. Sea salt should never be "well-roasted." Temperatures above 110° F. will destroy the sensitive minerals. However, since water and oil repel each other, only a dry salt will readily combine with the oil from the seeds.

diet are canceled without the penetrating action of salt and its minerals. Vegetables in their natural state, by nature, are lacking in sodium chloride. Vegetable juices and the water used for cooking grains readily dissolve salt crystals. Therefore, for proper assimilation, it is best to add salt in that form, rather than as finely ground when food is on the plate. Soy sauce may be used for a fancy flavor, but this much more expensive condiment is not necessary; besides, it is hard on the kidneys since all soy sauces available today are made with industrially-refined salt. Adding salt to vegetables as they are dry-sauteed releases their water, thus eliminating or reducing the amount of oil required for cooking. Once dissolved and ionized, the salt possesses a definite reactivity, has full electromagnetic capabilities, and passes more easily into the large colon where it will have a sanitizing effect.

There are times at the onset or in the early development of an illness when extra salting of food, for a strictly limited period — no more than three days, salt *is* powerful medicine — will effectively counteract an illness. This seemingly drastic measure does not truly constitute an excess of salt intake, due to the short duration. Everyone's tolerance and need for salt varies according to climate, activity, age, sex, and condition of health. Alcohol, vinegar, citrus, and other acid fruits readily dissolve the cohesive minerals in our body and cause a displacement of these mainly to joints and articulations, creating arthritic condition and skeletal malformation diseases.

A past history of having eaten unsalted vegetables/grains or consuming them with too little salt, especially refined salt, ends up by triggering a mechanism that instinctively pushes one to excess consumption in order to rectify this de-mineralization. Compounded by the sizeable amount of liquid inherently imbibed in vegetarian diets, and lacking the proper salt, the excess is not easily eliminated.

This not only creates a sudden excess of sodium and bloating, but due to kidney malfunction, these wet green leafy diets often cause further expansion of the belly and poor assimilation. If at first these diets seem to effect a short-term cleansing, they are, in the long run, of no benefit to the consumer. The goal of proper eating is ultimately to achieve a steady and stabilized harmony, and here, natural salt is the grounding crystal catalyst of excellence.

Beware of Crude-grade
Gray Salt from Refineries

Could a crude (dirty) unrefined salt, such as one would gather just before bulldozing by the giant refineries, be used? This is the kind that is slowly air-dried for as much as five years in the commercial salt fields of very polluted bays, it is then gathered mechanically and vacuum-processed. No amount of cleaning will make this crude salt safe as a food.

In recent years, motivated by the desire to obtain an unrefined salt, people have gathered and then dry-roasted that tainted, un-refined salt until it turns still darker, thinking that such a step would be enough to cleanse the salt of its industrial impurities. Such a practice is quite dangerous since no home process will ever effectively remove the poisonous elements of crude bay salt, much less eliminate the heavy metals: lead, cadmium, mercury, etc. Raw crude salt from bay side industrial ponds, even after being oven or pan dried, could never be made safe for human consumption.

Salt To Correct Sugar Addiction?

Sodium must be present in the digestive system in order for vegetal or even animal proteins to be transformed and absorbed. When the stomach contains a sufficient amount of hydrochloric acid, it properly digests the glucides of cereal grains and breaks down the fibers of vegetables. Salt is also required to emulsify fats and oils in order for them to be digestible. Hydrochloric acid is produced only if chlorine is present in the right ratio; this can be assured only if natural sea salt is used. For some people, eating whole grains sometimes causes an excessive, unnatural craving for sweets or "sweet and oily" desserts. This cancels the effectiveness of a grain diet, but when the cause is known the problem can easily be corrected. The glucides contained in grains signal to the digestive system that a form of sugar is being chewed and will soon reach the stomach for processing. But without any salt, too little of it, or especially a poor quality salt, these glucides do not transform at all. The body is completely denied the sugars it normally receives from this food, causing a drastic deficiency and the subsequent craving for sweets. The same salt deficiency also blocks the emulsifying of oil normally supplied adequately by the oil in the germ of whole cereals. This will cause one to use excess oil or to crave oily or butter-rich desserts even after a balanced whole grain meal.

Fermentation/Smart Fast Foods

The fermentation of vegetables (sauerkraut, pickles, kim'chee, pickles); grains (sourdough bread, kvass, kiesiel, kisra, koji); beans (miso, natto, tempeh) and fish are experiencing renewed interest. The savings in refrigeration costs alone would warrant the return to a safer, saner and more savory taste.

As the world's fastest and best quality foods, these are always ready to be consumed, cold or hot. Ancient traditional cookbooks almost never mentioned fermented fast foods for the simple reason that those cookbooks were written for the rich and famous. Reading these older texts, one gets the idea that our ancestors spent a great amount of time preparing those fancy and elaborate meals. The truth is elsewhere: simple folks who toiled in the fields for long hours, had need for quickly fixed moveable-feast style lunches to be consumed as the pickers and gleaners worked in the furrows. These foods often had to stand all morning long in the heat of harvest without the benefit of refrigeration.

Our fermented foods were created for just that purpose: Conservation without refrigeration and ready to serve quickly in the field or at the evening table. Sour dough breads, pickled olives, kippered herrings and anchovies, lacto-fermented vegetables and beans and sometimes yoghurt or cheese were the everyday fare that varied only slightly with the seasons.

A properly elaborated sourdough loaf acquires an unsurpassed taste and an aroma that no cracker or porridge can ever match. Sauerkraut achieves a succulent gourmet savor that cole-slaw never reaches. If you once taste Normandy country farm butter, churned from aged fermented sour cream, you will never be happy with raw cream butter.

These stable and satisfying basic foods owed their stability and superior taste to the miracle of microorganisms. These are not just smart biological living organisms but are also, the most talented high-quality fast-food chefs. The way they enhance all foods they treat is revealed in the root of their latin name, ferment comes from "fevere," to boil, and when one watches the brewing bubbly carbon dioxide gas that issues from the fermentation process, the food effectively appears to boil.

Added benefits offered by fermented foods are so numerous that we can only enumerate them here, since that topic is covered in detail in our soon to be released bread book.

1. Fermented foods gain in nutritive value over the same unfermented staple.
2. Fermentation neutralizes certain toxins.
3. Natural but unsafe counter-nutritive substances are broken

down and made harmless by fermentation, some of these are:

Saponin and trypsin: in soy beans and soy extracts
Phytic acid: in cereal grains and beans
Linamarin glucoside: in manioc (cassava) and tapioca
Aflatoxin: in peanuts and soy beans
Nitrosamine and nitrite: in fried fat of fish and meat

4. Fermentation can also pre-digest cereal grains, beans and milk products.

From all of the above, it is clear that mere sodium chloride — refined pickling or bakery salt — cannot correctly preserve and ferment foods while perfecting their taste. Ferments are alive and a complete salt, endowed with all macro-nutrients and trace elements, is necessary to ensure the propagation of harmonious, live friendly bacteria. Several pickle and miso makers and beer and soy sauce brewers as well as bakers have already recognized the wisdom of converting their operation to a natural fermentation utilizing the Celtic natural ocean salt. It stands to reason that magnesium-rich salts (about 0.7% in Celtic sea salt) are required to attract and nourish the right ferments and create the optimum environment for harmonious growth and fermentation.

The percentage of salt to be used is based on the weight of vegetables plus that of water for pickling. In baking it is calculated on the weight of the flour plus the water and starter combined. In the case of non-yeast natural fermentation for bread making, the amount of Celtic salt used is slightly less than one percent for whole-grain breads and up to 1½% for white bread. The higher quantity makes up for the missing minerals removed with the bran and the germ when using white flour. In all fermentations, the important advantage of keeping fresh without refrigeration for a long time (conservation) is achieved by the development of lactic acid and not

by the quantity of salt. In actual practice, the ideal quantity of salt for any lacto-fermented preparation is one half pound of salt for each 100 lbs of beans, vegetable or grain, or one half of 1%.

Making Mother Liquor

Fill a long, narrow cotton bag (10" x 24") with the whole original 22-pound bag of Celtic ocean salt. Tie a string around the neck of the cloth bag and dip it briefly in water (3 minutes). Hang the bag above a wide earthenware bowl (about 1 gallon capacity). Allow the mother liquor concentrate to drip into the container below. Store this cloudy-white liquid concentrate in a dark glass jar. Mother Liquor has numerous therapeutic uses, to cleanse wounds, baths (thalasso-therapy) and healing compresses. (The 1967 International Medical Congress of Cannes reported successful cures for no less than 600 different illnesses for this mother liquor water, from allergies to rickets to rheumatic fever).

The remaining wet salt from the cloth bag is poured on a large, clean, unpainted wooden surface or flat woven basket. Spread thinly and allow to dry in the sun for one hour to one whole day. Protect from dust or moisture and take the mats or boards inside at dusk. Storing the sun-redried salt in glass containers prevents moisture absorption. This salt, which has been briefly separated from its mother liquor and then sun-energized and re-crystallized, is whiter but still contains most of its valuable trace elements and macro-nutrients, it is still much more biologically active and effective.

It is not recommended to further pan-roast or oven dry this natural salt. If this salt is to be crushed with sesame seeds or ground for use in a shaker, drying in a warm cast iron pan only to the point of moisture removal is best. To make fine ground Celtic, flower of ocean or this salt much more free-running, mix in a few grains of parched rice in the shaker as a natural desiccant.

9

Iodine Laden Sea Breezes
and Iodized Salt

T HE absence of iodine in food intake is known to be a cause of goiter, a pathological state of thyroidal overdevelopment and malfunction. The thyroid gland does not secrete enough hormones and enlarges to compensate for its inadequate secretion. In actuality, the disease is caused by a deficiency of several minerals in the organism rather than by a lack of the single iodine element. In a commendable effort at compensating for the total lack of iodine in white table salt, the Food and Drug Administration spells out the quantity of supplemented iodine[1] that must be added to refined salt.

---

1. Added in the form of inorganic potassium iodide or sodium iodide, this is a quick "fix" that cannot adequately supply the starved glandular tissues, because either of these iodide salts leave the organism in as little as 20 minutes. In order to stabilize the volatile iodide compound, dextrose is added which turns the iodized salt an eerie purplish cast. A third additive, a bleaching agent, rectifies this unappetizing color shift and so consumers unknowingly consume two extra chemicals when purchasing "iodized salt."

Their rule is based on a minimum daily requirement (M.D.R.) not exceeding 0.15 milligrams, based on an average intake of 21 grams of salt per day. This M.D.R. translates into 7 milligrams of added iodine per kilo (2.204 lbs.) of white table salt.

The iodine-rich air near the seashore or around tidal waters liberates, by aerosolization (finely atomized sea spray or spin-drift), a sizeable amount of organic and beneficial iodine. The concentration of iodine carried in coastal air by this spin-drift spray is highest in winter, and is at maximum levels above deep ocean waters. Residents of countries and states that are far from the sea and thus without direct contact with marine air suffer from iodine deficiencies. In those areas, iodine is arbitrarily added to white commercial table salt for human consumption and also to the ration fed to pigs, chicken, and cattle.

A country where the problem of goiter exists on an even wider scale than in the U.S. central plains somehow arrived at a dosage of 6 milligrams daily (280 milligram/kilo), or about 40 times the amount added to iodized U.S. salt. In spite of these extreme corrective measures, Switzerland experiences numerous thyroidal complications. The widespread use of either Swiss-type iodized salt, or the lower-level iodine enriched U.S. salt, still does not prevent specific thyroid malfunctions. These are: hyperactivity of the autonomic nervous system, excessive secretion of thyroid hormone; increased cardiac output; obesity; low vitality; fragile teeth and bones; autoimmune diseases; inability to think logically; cretinism; paralysis of the sex organs; and, in women, abnormal development of the mammary glands.

The reason given by the refiners for adding more in refined salt than nature originally puts into natural sea salt is that endemic goiter (hyperplasia of the thyroid gland) can only be remedied by extra amounts of added iodine. There is mounting evidence that the inorganic form of iodine[1] added to refined white table salt, in any concentration, does not decrease goiter incidence. The iodine, added in this artificial and excessive way, passes in the urine within 20 minutes and all of it will have left the body within 24 hours. No research was ever made on the very real harm done by excessive doses of this artificially added iodine.

The Natural Way

The healing properties of iodine-rich marine products were known and used extensively for treating goiter well before iodine was isolated and discovered. Around 1500 B.C. the Greeks ate charred sea sponges and drank seaweed teas; later, both of these remedies were prescribed for the treatment of goiter by a Chinese physician, Ke-Hung, who lived 281–361 A.D. The Chinese pharmacopoeia in the eighth century A.D. listed no less than 27 different prescriptions for the treatment of goiter, all of them using forms of sea algae and other products of the sea. Modern medicine discovered that iodine was a prime constituent of the thyroid gland in 1895, and the thyroid hormone, thyroxin, was first isolated in 1914. In the first enthusiasm of discovery, all sorts of foods—human and livestock—were supplemented with quantities of iodine totally out of proportion to the needs of the human or animal thyroid gland. Today, the salt refiners, misguided by the medical establishment, continue this practice. Seventy-five years later, such overdoses continue unabated (an average of 30 to 1200 times the dosage that occurs in natural Celtic ocean salt). Iodine supplementation in inorganic form (such as through iodized table salt or tablets) is responsible for many vague glandular "borderline" symptoms without actual pathology.

While small amounts of iodine are found in the blood, nerves,

---

1. Potassium iodide is most often used.

and other organs, most of the body's iodine is present in the thyroid, ovaries, and uterus, with women appearing to require a somewhat larger supplemental dosage than men. The principal periods of increased demand for iodine are during puberty, pregnancy and menopause or when infection or great stress of the body's functions occur. Further, the iodine element is involved in the metabolism of calcium and phosphorus and the proper absorption of the complex carbohydrates. Essential for physical and mental development, the iodine salts are initially absorbed in the intestine. It is there that the free iodine is bound in thyroxine and can then migrate to all body cells. Since it does not remain in the blood supply for any length of time, daily replenishment by minute amounts of organic iodine is vital. This transient form of iodine is called "protein-bound iodine." That very minute but precise amount required daily can be much more easily met by Celtic unrefined ocean salts. The quantity of chemical iodine added to white table salt, cattle feed or lick blocks now varies between 10 and 400 milligrams per kilogram. The actual supplementation in food-grade iodized salt is 1 part of sodium iodide to every 100,000 parts of sodium chloride.[1]

An excess of iodine in any diet is as detrimental as a lack of it. Such an excessive dosage, beyond the possibility of causing hypoplasia (underdevelopment) of the thyroid, may affect many hormonal and metabolic functions. Iodine enters into the making of two hormones secreted by the thyroid gland: thyroxin and tetra-iodothyronine (T_4). Both of these play an important part in numerous metabolic functions, more specifically in regulating body temperature and building resistance to cold.

The organic forms of iodine as found in algae, sea plants and

---

1. Natural sun-dried Celtic gray sea salt contains 0.35 mgr. of complex organic iodine salts per kilo of salt crystals, or 30 to 1200 times *less* than the refined white "enriched" iodized salt.

fish remain in the body fluids an average of 48 hours with traces of iodine still actively at work in the body for several weeks afterwards. When any salt is artificially heated or even partially refined by processing such as boiling, kiln-drying or electrolysis, it loses all of its highly volatile iodine and even the more stable micro-algal iodine as well. Not a trace of either kind remains.

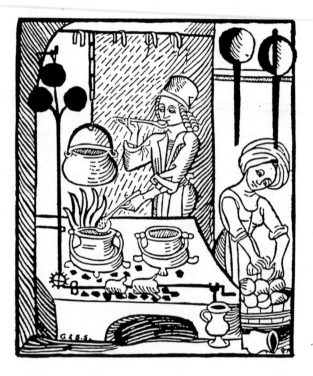

10

How Nature
Makes Iodine

G RANITE rocks release part of their tin content to the stems and roots of most sea vegetation, while the leaves of these plants collect lithium from sea water. In November the sea-weeds die and release the combination—Tin + Lithium = Iodine — into the oceans. One ton of seawater will yield only a few milligrams of iodine, while about 2 milligrams of iodine are found in each kilo of natural ocean salt. But iodine is volatile and after a year of storage, only 0.4 milligrams, or less than one fifth of the original iodine quantity, remain in one kilogram of sun-dried sea salt. Slightly more passes into the salt if it contains some clay particles; these ionize, fix and retain the iodine. At the seashore, most of the iodine aerosolizes into marine air and becomes part of the sea breeze and moist spray coming from the crests of the waves. These aerosolized trace elements penetrates several miles inland unless city or industrial pollutants near the coast block their progress from the coast.

Ocean salt, naturally sun-dried, tenaciously retains a sizeable amount of moisture. This dries out only if the salt is subjected to the extreme heat of refinery kilns or saltmaker's ovens. While magnesium salts are the major chemical elements preserved by this moisture, the sun-formed whole salt crystals hold many more trace elements securely, among them the valuable organic iodine compounds. Additionally, beneficial microscopic particles of phytoplankton and algal organisms are trapped within the Celtic sea salt, endowing the crystals with additional vegetal quality iodine.

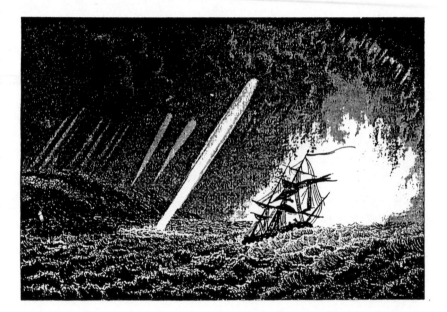

11

Radiation Fallout Protection

T HE daily use of natural gray Celtic sea salt protects the user by neutralizing fallout radiation exposure because it supplies organic iodine to the entire glandular network. The new science of microchemistry[1] has proven that several specific trace elements protect the internal organs from artificial radiation, and that these oligo-elements are most effective at micro-doses. In life-threatening situations such as direct exposure to atomic radiation, potassium iodide tablets are prescribed in an attempt to quickly saturate the thyroid. It is hoped that this massive and sudden supplementation can save lives by competing with and serving to clear the radioactive iodine that concentrate in the thyroid after exposure to an atomic blast. The prescribed potassium iodine forces the radioactive iodine

---

1. A relatively new facet of biological medicine, microchemistry shows that the healing of a number of illnesses depends directly on the presence and action of metallic ions in the body: magnesium, iodine, iron and sodium, at the molecular scale.

to leave the body. This medical theory speculates that, as the tablets flush the endocrinal system, the lethal effect of radioactive iodine will be checked. Dr. William Weston, while an official in the United States Department of Public Health, stated that the organically bound iodine of foodstuffs (land-based algae, seaweeds, crabs, oysters, lobsters, shrimps, etc.) is far more effective because it is slowly released into the body. Artificially supplemented iodine is worthless because it passes too quickly into the urine within as little as twenty minutes. A better way to prepare against the eventuality of atomic fallout is to build a strong immune terrain ahead of time by simply using real sea salt daily since it alone supplies the highest possible level of organic iodine. The fixing capabilities of the clay stabilize the iodine level at 800 parts per million, which is more than half of the iodine of sea water. While iodine is volatile and some of it escapes into the atmosphere, the loss is minimized because crystallization is completed in less than 12 hours. In the industrial exploitation of salt, the salty brine stagnates from a few months to as much as three years in the ponds and all of the iodine is already evaporated in the crude stage well before further loss is inflicted before the refining process is even begun.

It takes 30 liters (8 gallons) of sea water to produce one kilogram of natural Celtic salt crystals.[1] In the original liquid form of those 30 liters, the iodine content is on the order of 1500 parts per million. Soil and crops near coastlines are richer in organic iodine than those inland. Eating seaweeds, shore-grown vegetables or tideland saltwort[2] will supply as much as 100 milligrams of iodine per serving.

---

1. If totally refined salt is the goal, 40 liters (10.8 gallons) must be processed to obtain one kilo (2.204 lbs.) of pure sodium chloride (white table salt.)

2. Saltwort are any of the various plants of sea beaches, salt marshes and alkaline regions, especially of the genus Salsola, as Salsola Kali, a bushy plant having prickly leaves, or of the genus Salicornia.

The latest findings in biology demonstrate that natural Celtic ocean salts contain not only organic iodine compounds but that those levels are reinforced by the presence of iodine-bearing microscopic algal and phytoplankton organisms that add organic quality iodine to these salts. If the natural moisture in salt is forced-out or if it is stored in too hot an area, the salt will lose both of these iodine forms. Therefore, it is always wise to purchase natural Celtic ocean salt, a moist salt and to protect its humidity by always storing it in a cool and dark place.

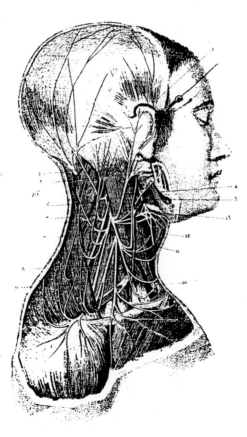

12

Sex, Salt and Your Kidneys

D OES the quality of salt affect sexuality, and if so, how does it alter this? There most definitely is a correlation between salt quality and sexual harmonious maturity, indeed, a very strong one. Kidney failure in both men and women that occurs due to nephron breakdown is very common today. Insoluble crystals of hemoglobin form in these nephrons and are the cause of the failure. The cortical hormones, secreted by the adrenal cortex, literally program both man's and woman's sexual instinct by improving the quality of the energy of the gonads. When these hormones are adequately and sufficiently secreted, it assures that friendship and sentimental warmth will be experienced toward all of humanity, and that a caring, loving feeling for the opposite sex unfolds as an intuitive experience. Salt is the catalyst that helps to develop a harmonious sexual character; its subtle essence plays a major role in defining and affirming the characteristics in both sexes.

The male, biologically and traditionally, has been the initiator and the female the receptor. To maintain that enterprising trait, men instinctively consume slightly more salt than women. The additional salt also serves to balance the male glandular functions, since men have more expanded constitutions. This is evidenced by the male larger and external sexual organs.

Man, by intuition, has to consume slightly more salt than the female, this use to help develop in him the "provider" trait necessary to hunt and gather food, to initiate relationships, and, if need be, to defend his mate and family. But it is in the area of male virility and sexual character that two of the components of the hormone corti- sone really accomplish great changes. Androsterone and testosterone both help regulate the size of the genitalia, develop good sexual instinct and response, maintain the deeper tones of the male voice and develop good sexual instinct and response. These two substances are also responsible for bulkier skeletal development, heavier bone formation, and genuine virility.

The secretions of the adrenals and the pituitary gland are measurably curtailed when refined salt is used. Vasopressin or ADH and the hormone cortisol that are vital to assure optimum sexual functions are no longer secreted when white table salt is the condiment. These sexual malfunctions, added to the retention of body fluids (caused by the absence of magnesium salts in refined salt), can create a combination that destroys sexual functions and sensitive response.

The adrenal glands, sometimes called the glands of combat, secrete masculine motivators and regulators, circulating them in the system. Any muscular activity; average, normal and daily stress; as well as salty or high protein foods —whether from animal or vegetable origin —tend to stimulate the male adrenal cortex in a positive manner. Uncommon stress however, that which upsets and harms the inner self, occurs only when the cortex becomes depleted by a lack of trace and macro-minerals in the food or by the excessive consumption of protein. It is this stress that is harmful because it creates cruel and careless behavior, the kind of uncontrollable emotions that lead to disharmony, vehement strife and passionate crimes.

What Is the Effect of Refined Salt on Women ?

When trace minerals are absent from the salt a woman uses, ACTH, the adrenocorticotropic hormone, begins to affect all her glands, from the pituitary to the adrenal cortex. These strong male hormones, the androgens, become overpowering and tend to change female characteristics into male aggressive traits by stimulating the adrenal cortex. There are uniquely feminine internal secretions of the ovaries: the estrogens, the luteins, and the folliculins; when these are replaced by the male androgens, the exquisite femininity. disappears. This can all be caused by the use of white refined salt.

Women are highly intuitive by nature. In order to maintain this trait, their food and their salt need to be selected differently than for men. Flower of Ocean Celtic is an ideal feminine salt. Women become unhappy when they take too much meat, fish, cheese or refined salt. When they do indulge in these, women will often suffer from menstrual irregularities. If they love at all they usually choose men with passive, obedient traits, or other women, often the kind that also are more submissive. Their delicate feminine balance is lost due to the taking of food and salt that are contrary to the intuitive character of their sex.

The reproductive system functions as well as a calm and harmonious mood in both men and women are influenced and determined by the health of the kidneys. A breakdown in the gonad performance is caused by a failure of the kidneys.

The kidneys are very efficient filtration organs. Without the continuous cleansing that they provide, the blood would become so toxic that a person would die in a matter of days. It is because of their busy schedule that they are often tired and overtaxed.

Refined salt produces pain, aches or tightness in the back, indicating a problem in the kidney function. Nearly everyone who uses refined salt experiences this at some time or another, and a stepped-up liquid intake relieves the problem only very briefly. This only compounds the problem, since the kidneys now have a greater volume of water as well as hard refined salt in the form of kidney stones (see "Salt and Healing" in the next chapter) to contend with and try to eliminate. This overwork makes them weaker, resulting in a lowering of sexual energy in both women and men.

Natural salt allows liquids to freely cross body membranes, the kidney's glomerulus and blood vessel walls. Whenever the sodium chloride concentration rises in the blood, the water in the neighboring tissues is attracted to that salt-rich blood; then, if they are functioning properly, the kidneys remove the saline fluids easily. Refined salt does not allow this free crossing of liquids and minerals, and causes accumulated fluids to stagnate in joints, producing edema and chronic kidney problems.

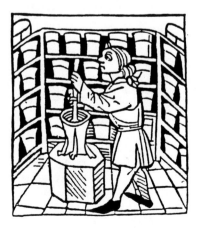

13

Salt Phobia

MANY persons are actually unable to tolerate salty foods at all. That intolerance affects the quality of their health as well as their character. Lacking warmth and affection, these persons remain unhappy. This stems from any of the following causes:

1. A high salt concentration remaining in tissues and fluids, due to salt plus meat consumption;
2. Kidneys that have become weak or failed to function;
3. Conditioned judgment—the person blames the food, the cook, the water but refuses to recognize his or her condition.

Biology states that excess salt collects in tissues and body fluids. However, only refined salt will cause this problem. Natural Celtic salt does not accumulate in the tissues; the magnesium salts will eliminate sodium chloride after it has performed its important jobs of acid-base balance, cell permeability and muscle contractibility. If an excess of natural salt is ingested, then the intake of water is automatically increased by a thirst that craves liquids. The quantity of salt above that which is needed by the body is automatically rejected by the body, but much more easily if natural salt is used. An unbalanced diet or malfunctioning kidneys are much lesser causes of salt retention. An oversalted condition can become chronic when blood vessel walls are shut tightly by the hardness of refined salt. The disruption of sexual functions is only a warning signal announcing impending illnesses such as urinary tract infections, Addison's disease, kidney cancer or albumen in the urine.

Addison's disease is a condition of adrenal deficiency. Some of the symptoms are: abnormal cravings for more salt; weak sex drive; gradual darkening of the skin and mucus membranes; and puffiness of face and jaw. This illness has been described as tuberculosis of the adrenals. In symptomatic medicine, it is treated by a steady regimen of hormone injections.

These medications create high blood pressure due to fluid retention made worse by the use of refined salt. They also cause the toxins of these drug and hormone injections to concentrate and stagnate in the body which inevitably results in vulnerability to more disease.

One of the major functions of the adrenal cortex is to secrete the hormone cortisone, sodium being a mineral vitally needed for human metabolism, a healthy adrenal cortex prevents the unwarranted elimination of sodium salts. This, together with aldosterone, regulates and balances salt and water throughout the body. Natural cortisone has many other functions, from changing protein into glucides and changing food into cells, to preventing inflammation.

Salt and Healing

Celtic sea salt has countless medicinal uses. It can help in correcting excess acidity; restoring good digestion; relieving allergies and skin diseases; and preventing many forms of cancer. Natural salt provides a steady boost in cellular energy and gives the body a heightened resistance to infections and bacterial diseases. Lima Ohsawa, macrobiotic healer in Japan, has emphatically stated many times, "If you cook your vegetables without salt, you will never cure any illness." Refined salt has lost its ionic, electrolytic, positive and negative charge properties. It is that particular bio-electronics quality which makes Celtic ocean salt a healing element and a vital, necessary added ingredient in any vegetarian diet.

Natural sea salt dried by the sun's rays contains elements that enhance the human organism by their radioactive properties. It is possible to follow the path of radio calcium as it heads straight to the site of a bone fracture or lesion of an organ upon entering the body. Other radioactive isotopes work in the same manner, such as radio-manganese, radio-phosphorus, or radio-magnesium.

These simple isotopes are led, ionically and electronically, in a straight pathway through the body to their required destination, unerringly reaching the spot where they are needed most. They not only perform such mechanical tasks as bone fracture mending, but are also able to totally restore chronic organic malfunctions and correct aberrant mental conditions.

The 70-plus trace elements have definite triggering actions on the body's various functions, feeding the organs with a specific amount —measurable in parts per million—of elements that help to eliminate or prevent disease. Biomedical research has, for years, recognized that a number of illnesses are directly preventable by the action of metallic ions in the organism such as magnesium, calcium, iron, sodium, and potassium.

Isolating and administering these elements in the form of mineral supplements is a popular method of treatment whenever a deficiency is diagnosed by hair, nail, body fluid, or fecal analysis. Minerals work in conjunction with each other, and they cannot work to heal when their concentration is increased disproportionately beyond the level of parts per million. Even in a dosage that consists in taking just one tablet of mineral supplementation, the effect can be toxic by upsetting the balance of minerals rather than beneficial.

Micro-dosages such as the magnesium salts, as they exist in naturally sun-dried sea salt, which average about .75% of the total ocean solids, are essential for the electrical breakdown of nutrients. As enzyme activators and controllers of energy transfer in living cells, magnesium salts are also catalysts for carbohydrate metabolism and chemical reactions in the body. They regulate bone and brain development, blood plasma, and dissolve calcium oxalate deposits, more commonly called kidney stones. If, as in boiled salt, the magnesium salts are lacking or insufficient (less than one half of one percent), kidney stones will form.

Taking a salt containing between half and three-quarters of 1% of magnesium salt prevents the formation of kidney stones, or dissolves those already formed. Magnesium salts in excess of 3% of total solids in salt will, on the other hand, create hardening of the joints and extreme arthritis. Phosphorus is present in natural sea salt also in micro-amounts, that of a period followed by four zeroes and then four sixes (0.00006666). Phosphorus salt compounds initiate and renew bone material which in turn maintain ionic blood composition. They regulate hydrogen ion concentration and vitamin absorption in tissue, and prevent rickets and osteoporosis.

When is it necessary to take in more salt than a normal dose? In the case of hemorrhage, severe burns, violent physical trauma, acute infection, shock from an illness, surgical intervention, or if very deep emotional turmoil occurs, there is an immediate requirement for extra potassium. This is best met by a salt solution made directly from a natural light gray Celtic sea salt. This restores the potassium in the inner cell through the process of transmutation from sodium.[1]

---

1. See C. Louis Kervran, *Biological Transmutations*, trans. Michel Abhesera (Magalia, Calif.: Happiness Press, 1988).

Proper balance in the body is achieved by maintaining a relatively high potassium content inside the cell and a relatively high sodium concentration outside the cell. When these elements are in excess, this reestablishment of balance can occur in many ways: through urine, sweat, tears, feces, or even vomiting.

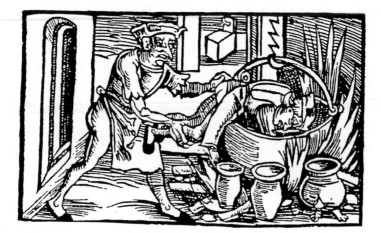

14

The Roots of
Human Wisdom

ANCIENT peoples had powers which we have lost for the most part. For example, the Egyptian pyramids reveal wonders of mathematical and technological intelligence that we would be hard put to duplicate even with modern engineering techniques. Thus the creators of the pyramids, and other advanced ancient civilizations, could hardly be called primitive.

Minerals from land masses have constantly been washed into the sea by the action of streams and rains. The ancients knew that all human essences after death similarly flowed into the sea, brought there from the immortal spirit of the departed, either by runoffs, rains or floods, and that these essences of human enlightenment could, in a specific way, be passed on to the following generations. The men and women of prehistoric times lived in a very different state of consciousness and moved within cosmic forces, which endowed them with strength and wisdom far beyond our own.

Their manner of passing this legacy was accomplished by the rite of passage at birth that consisted of placing a few moist crystals of sea salt on the tongue of the initiate to insure that the recipient would grow righteous, pure, and wise, by the powers thus inherited from their ancestors, as well as from God and the akashic records.[1] This ritual is still part of the baptismal ceremonies today.

It would appear, therefore, that the human hunger for salt reaches far deeper than a simple biochemical need. It is instinct that compels us to consume the salt extracted from the fluid element of the planet's great cauldron. This practice connects us directly with our ancestors' wealth of experience and wisdom. This instinct moves us to prefer salt from the sea over that from land mines; it also seems that, when given the choice, we intuitively choose whole natural ocean salt over the refined. This sum total of human character and knowledge is transferred to us only by the salt and not by any other sea product: fish, plankton or seaweeds, because salt alone crosses the barrier of the cell membrane and triggers a hormone-cell homing mechanism that, before materialism, was transmitted to human genes through air- and waterborne pheromones.[2]

Insects, fishes and mammals are still following their forebear's gene waves or pheromones but humans have lost this trait, possibly due to their alienation from natural elements and the environment. In former times, our link with the watery part of the planet may have been accomplished through our internal saline fluids due to their similarity to sea water. Our pheromonal mechanism appears to be derived from an encoding trapped within the moist crystal

---

1. A veiled memory of all events, thoughts and experiences that have inspired and guided humankind since the beginning of time; encoded in a fluid ether that exists beyond the range of human material senses and reputedly accessible only to certain chosen individuals.

2. A chemical used in intraspecific communication between animals, it triggers their guidance mechanism. Pheromones are freely dispersed in their environment, the sea for fishes and dolphins, in the air as scented guideposts or laid down on earth trail for insects and mammals.

structure of natural sea salt, the pilot that directs our genetic cells. The amino acids of the microflora (micro-algae) within the crystals are transported to the core of our cells by our own internal saline solution. The nitrogen, mineralized by the salt's fixing agents, is absorbed by the aminity function that interacts with an algae-rich environment. This creates a new molecule, an amino acid that is intimately bonded to life by its evolutionary characteristic: It appears sometimes as acid or alkaline, depending on the circumstances. Regular molecules do not possess this ability to change from acid to alkaline and vice versa. This capability, called amphoteric quality,[1] is retained for as long as the salt crystal remains moist. The minute quantities of guidepost molecules, once regrouped in our body, constitute an action command post formed by a group of hormones, vitamins and diastases.

Within salt crystals, certain simple elements exist that enhance genes. These are simple isotopes[2] that are led ionically and guided in a straight pathway to their planned destination. These isotopes work not only to correct genetic errors and mental aberrations but also, in some well-documented cases, are capable of completing such mechanical tasks as mending bones.

Finally, various trace elements found only in naturally crystallized salt can act positively by their reactive properties on the human organism. It is possible to track the rebuilding process of radio-calcium in the bone-rebuilding process mentioned above, but it has been discovered that other radio isotopes work in the same manner. Within a salt solution, made from natural crystals, unheated and diluted to an isotonic concentration—i.e., having the same osmotic pressure

---

1. Said of a substance that reacts with both acids and bases, acting as an acid in the presence of a base and as a base in the presence of an acid.

2. Two or more atomic species of the same chemical element having different atomic masses.

as blood serum—one can detect the presence of radio-manganese, radio-iron, radio-phosphorus, etc., that is to say: radioactive macro-elements as well as radioactive trace elements.

In order for a salt to be endowed with this beneficial radioactivity, it must be harvested from salt flats along coastlines that are in direct linkage with oceanic fields that are favored with both upwellings and cosmic ionization.

At depths greater than 200 feet, sea water is most receptive to cosmic ionization. Cosmic rays are known to penetrate and ionize the ocean layers at optimum levels of 240 feet. (Measured with Geiger counter by Schmitt.)

Upwelling occurs where lighter-gravity water meets heavier water; this meeting creates strong kinetic up and down movements that bring organic and mineral nutrients to the upper layers of the sea where the largest concentration of marine life thrives. This has a direct influence on the quality of radioactive and pheromonal manifestation.

Oceans Less Polluted Than Land Areas

Numerous marine biologists have noted the seemingly untarnished and constant state of purity of sea water, in spite of its coastlines' pollution. We are witnessing here a surprising phenomenon that yields some remarkable facts.

Experiments carried out in France by M. Le Foch demonstrate that sea water contains some definitely antiseptic constituents dispersed in the total phyto-marine medium. These destroy bacteria. Heavily polluted river water shows that its bulk of bacteria die the moment they enter the sea, the oceans behave as if they were a completely self-cleaning environment, since the majority of coliform bacilli in sewage cannot be traced or found a few miles out at sea. While this fact alone will not reassure us on the state of the planet, an in vitro test quickly proves that pathogenic bacteria can only survive for a short time in the presence of living sea water. This property of destroying bacilli remains effective only as long as that sea water is not stored in bottles, or as long as the salt is not industrially dried.

Because of the unique ability of the ocean to absorb, neutralize and clean much of the man-made pollution, nothing of an injurious nature can survive in the great cauldron; what remains is the widest collection of all the minerals that exist on the planet, churning in living waters, as well as the deepest, wisest and most awesome pool of human memory, the akashic record which is the eternal storage of spiritual life from humanity's past.

By their very saline content, all oceans of the world offer the strongest protection against atomic radiation and fallout that humankind has available. The power to neutralize radiation comes not just from the high percentage of sodium chloride in the sea but also from the 16% of other salt compounds present in unrefined salt. It is the combination of all these mineral compounds in a symbiotic mix that gives the strongest protection to the consumers. Washed or artificially dried salt does not offer the same defense since the vital trace elements have disappeared.

The next criterion to be applied, when looking for cleanliness, is the geographic location of the salt flats. A survey of the Brittany coast shows no shipping lanes (it is a long way from the English Channel and the Normandy coastline), no oil rigs or terminals, or any large towns anywhere near the installations. The fast and discriminating method used for harvesting also contributes to a cleaner salt since the moving fresh brine changes into crystals within a day.

Our family visits the Celtic salt marshes in Brittany an average of once every two years and cover the four and a half million acres of the entire peninsula. Our observations have reassured us that the cleanliness and unpolluted quality of sea water of that particular coast continues to offer the safest protection against much of the pollution.

Alchemy and Salt

S ALT is the sublimation of the oceans. Since human beginnings it has been the symbol for spiritual excellence, pristine purity, esteem, devotion and even immortality. Today, the powers of salt are still concealed from many, but to the serious contemporary alchemists, it is revealing certain of its vital secrets.

Alchemy was ushered into human consciousness by the need to discover the relationship of humans to the cosmos, but also to explore all of the ways this kinship could benefit humanity. It naturally pointed to the ocean as the strongest manifestation of astral influence on earth. Alchemy, since its inception, dealt with humanity's relationship to terrestrial nature and the phenomena of this planet's elements and oceans — and its sublimation into crystals of salt by the sun, or by fire in the alchemist's workshop. Salt was the pivotal mineral complex substance that warranted deep study and was considered as the primary of all transmutation elements. One of the most enlightened alchemists of our time, the late Professor **C. Louis Kervran**, discovered transmutation at low energy, and in his experiments he succeeded in transforming one chemical element into another. His scientific research and formulas have been hailed by the scientific establishment and he was a candidate for the Nobel Prize. Having discovered and elucidated this extraordinary transformational property of matter, Professor Kervran[1] brought alchemy to grudging recognition by modern physicists.

In the search for the Elixir of Immortality, the alchemists of ancient times studied the ageless sea and its awesome energy. When they solved the enigma, the secret was kept from the prying eyes of the common mortals. In a very tangible way, the rediscovery by Professor Kervran links us to the secret of immortality and reveals its prime source.

In the Western World, the objective of alchemy, which is called The Art, seems to have evolved from gold making to elixirs of immortality to simply superior medicine. Neither the first nor the last of these objectives appear ever to have been important in China. Chinese alchemy was consistent in its quest and there was no controversy among its practitioners; the elixir of life was their sole goal, and it varied only in the formulation of its prescription or perhaps only in the name used.

While Europe witnessed conflicts between advocates of herbal and chemical (i.e., mineral) pharmacy, China wholly accepted trace minerals from seawater as remedies; the latter physicians also added fermentations of briny salt pickles, salted sour plums,[2] and other salty fermentations as powerful and effective medicines.

---

1. Professor C. Louis Kervran, 1901–1983, Director of Conferences at Paris University. A French genius in biology and biochemistry. His biological trans-mutation hypothesis questions the very nature of substance by advancing the theory that elements as well as living systems can create new elements. Of Kervran's more than twenty books, only one is available in English: *Biological Transmutations* (Magalia, Calif.: Happiness Press, 1989).

2. See *The Ume Plum's Secrets*, by Dr. Moriyasu Ushio, M.D. (Magalia, Calif.: Happiness Press, 1988).

In Europe, conflicts arose between alchemists who favored the gold-making objectives and those who thought medicine should be their sole occupation. The Chinese always pursued the prolongation of life and the enhancement of its quality. Both alchemies, Oriental as well as Old World, have spent centuries studying how the use of morning dew creates "the gold of the thousandth dawn." The similarity between this and the aerosolization of ocean spray and of mother liquor shows that their search centered on recreating the noble essence of the ocean.

The secret of extracting the mother liquor (bitterns) from the just-forming salt crystals dates back to the Celts and the Druids. Known as "Eaux-mères" (literally "mother's waters" in French), these riches that salt farmers keep separate from the salt contained the essence of all minerals of this planet except for the sodium chloride. Bitter in taste, this mother liquor serves to enhance preserved vegetables such as sauerkraut and pickles, but it also was found to resonate to the human body's most complex chemical assemblage of essential minerals, the internal body fluids. When it is taken in its pristine state, mother liquor helps cure many illnesses caused by mineral deficiencies. It also effectively acts as a preventive against physical and mental disturbances.

Traditional bitterns, as those extracted by Celtic salt farmers today, retain all of the noble trace minerals because they are sublimated by the sun, not by the searing heat used in the flash crystallizers of today's industrial refineries. Bitterns can only be created from whole salt and ionized by the gentle action of the clay in the salt pans. Only these bitterns are truly healing. Natural bitterns steadily retain enough moisture to remain deliquescent, thus the name "Mother Liquor."

The industrial counterpart is also called "bitterns," but being a waste byproduct of the industrial exploitation of the ocean by the salt refining industry, it is a pale and anemic imitation of the natural mother liquor. Commercial refiners strip "crude and polluted salt" of all its noble elements which they sell elsewhere; what is left are the commercial bitterns sometimes used in tofu making and other Asian food preparations.

The method used for the making of natural and moist mother liquor at home is described in detail on page 33. The ancestral way of farming salt flats by the Celtic method is described in full detail in a 300-page book, available as a reprint, from the publisher.[1]

The secret of physical immortality or the Endless Prolongation of Life was the subject of serious study in ancient times. The successful experiments of many modern-day alchemists prove that it is not an unattainable goal: to wit, the late French scientist **Dr. Alexis Carrel** kept a chicken heart alive for over 37 years by having the pulsating heart in a solution of sea salt. Dr. Carrel voluntarily ended the experiment after a third of a century, having proven that living cells can have physical immortality.[2]

It is sea water's sublimation, the true light grey sea salt, which is the perfect symbiotic culture medium for living human cells. With a saltiness that is compatible with all body fluids, amniotic water as well as plasma, it could be the fluid substance that all alchemists sought as the regenerator of life or the philosopher's stone.

Jabi ibn Hayyan, a Muslim Sufi alchemist who lived from 720 to 800 A.D., in his *Summa Perfectionis Magisterii* mentions not only Regal Water but makes allusions to Lustral Water (or Lustrum: water

---

1. Although the large book is only available in the original French version, it constitutes such an important document that its details must be spread far and wide. Thus we have placed the book, *Paludiers de Guèrande* by P. Lemonier, in many safe places around the globe in order to preserve the craft for future generations. (Available from Happiness Press.)

2. See *Man, the Unknown* (1936) by Alexis Carrel.

for the rites of purification) as well. Both are forms of ocean water that shimmer and fluoresce due to the electromagnetically-charged particles and all of the precious chemical elements of life that it contains.

The Belgian historian **Henri Pirenne** observed that during the High Middle Ages, the entire coast of the Atlantic was deserted and the entire continent was thrown into a Dark Age of human under-development. Historians tell us that it was caused to a great extent by the lack of salt in the human diet, the flooding of all salt flats having disabled every salt farm along the coastlines of the Atlantic Ocean and the Mediterranean Sea. The whole of Europe, therefore, suffered from a salt famine that was to last almost 500 years. The daily average ration fell to less than 2 grams per person and caused many to die from dehydration and madness. The extent of the salt famine reported by Henri Pirenne caused human flesh to be sold on the open-air markets and created an epidemic of crazed people who, to replenish their salt, drank blood from the neck artery of the person they had just slain. Quick to exploit this desperate situation for their own gain, the rulers of Europe grabbed the remnants of the salt stock and exacted exorbitant salt taxes. Heavily burdened by tariffs and gabelles, common salt became a luxury but also caused mass population shifts and exodus, lured invaders and caused wars. Mined salt from the depths of the earth was substituted, but the lack of live and balanced trace elements in rock salt lowered the mental equilibrium and intellect level almost as much as the sheer absence of salt.

Only sea salt with its rich trace elements can insure the proper mental and body functions; without it these functions either slow down or stop altogether. For instance, the magnesium, bromide, and iodine salts are found in adequate concentration in the Celtic salts of Brittany, whereas the white refined salt, the mined salt, and those of the Great Salt Lake, the Red Sea and the Dead Sea contain these minerals in disharmony. When these trace elements begin to disappear from the human diet, mental and muscular fatigue set in, followed by depression, epilepsy, stress, impotence, frigidity and even folly.

The damages wreaked on humanity by the lack of salt for the five hundred years of the Dark Ages were considerable but today, in spite of an abundant consumption of pure white refined salt, this marasmus has returned in another form. Since only 7% of the total production of refined salt is used for food, salt refiners have supplied that same emasculated refined white chemical salt because it is cheap to harvest, ignoring the danger that it lowers the human psyche, only to satisfy the demands of an ever-growing chemical industry. Gradually during the past five centuries, salt merchants have mercilessly refined edible salt in order to extract from it the precious trace minerals: magnesium for the light alloys and the explosives; boron for anti-knock compounds and chemical fertilizers are just two examples. The biological demands of the human body require that the salt concentration in the blood and the body fluids be maintained at a constant level. If the body does not get enough salt, or consumes only the wrong (refined) quality, a hormonal mechanism compensates by reducing the excretion of salt in the urine and from sweat glands. But it cannot retain the totality of all body salts. On a completely salt-less diet, the body steadily loses small amounts of salt via the kidneys and perspiration. It then attempts to adjust to this by accelerating its secretion of water as well, so that the blood's salt concentration can be maintained at the level vital for survival. The result is a gradual desiccation, dehydration, of the body and finally death, often preceded by a loss of rational thinking — dementia or running amok. The organism literally dies of thirst.

In the case of lack of water to drink, the water is retained in order to maintain the salt concentration in the blood, but the hormonal control mechanism works in reverse. It tries to reduce the secretion of water and increase the salt secretion in order to maintain the correct salt level; nonetheless, the inevitable, irreducible water loss leads to death. In short, the body's normal craving for salt and for water strives toward the same vital need: a balanced and healthy saline internal fluid.

From the year 500 A.D. to the tenth century, making salt by any means became a necessity for survival and even the alchemists attempted to do it. However, compounding sea salt and duplicating the work of the great oceans of the world, which has taken billions of years, is, even for alchemists of old or medical blood lab workers of today, an impossible task. In the laboratories of the alchemists, the rarity and nobility of some of the micro substances created an even deeper respect for the mysterious natural ocean salt crystals.

The Emerald Tablet is no longer cryptic if the crystallization and subsequent sublimation of mother liquor from the sea salt crystals are studied and understood:

Separate the Earth from Fire, the subtle from the crude with much travail.

It rises from the Earth toward the sky, and immediately comes back on Earth where it gathers the force of superior and inferior creations. You will then have all the glory of the world and that is why all darkness will leave you.

The drinkable sea water called "Plasma of Quinton," —a name registered in 1907 by **René Quinton**, one of France's most renowned modern-day alchemists—is such a life-giving fluid that it dispels the darkness and gloom of sickness. It is still made today by a secret natural process. Unlike the approximation of the Ringer solution, still currently used in hospitals today, Quinton's plasma wholly duplicates the exact saline balance and restores the proper composition of human body fluids.

Quinton's Plasma continues to save lives as it has for the past 83 years. The biologist first successfully treated athrepsia with it and subsequently opened hundred of clinics throughout Europe, dispensed the precious plasma and won the battle for life over death in many other terminal ailments for thousand of patients.[1] Severe opposition from the ranks of modern medicine forced these clinics out of existence but today the serum is back and continues to quietly perpetuate the miraculous discovery of this latter-day alchemist.

The crisis that developed in all of Western Europe due to the flooding of the ancient salt flats by a phenomenon called "eustatic ebb and flow" saw the penetration of Arabic alchemy into Spain, then spreading to all of the Mediterranean world. Under Pope Sylvester II (who had read the Arabic alchemists' works), the newly imported alchemy established itself in its true realm: that of the technique of salvation, physical as well as moral. **C. G. Jung**, in his *Psychology and Alchemy*, sees alchemy as aiming to deliver the spark of eternal light from the abyss of the darkness of matter.

Mikhael Ivanov, who perpetuates in our time the flickering flame of Gnostic thought, symbolizes it in this way:

The blood of the Earth is Water, the Oceans are its Heart,
the vast planetary heart where plasmic blood is in abundance.
The rivers, lakes and streams are the arteries and the veins.
The lungs (much more extended than the heart) are the earth's
atmosphere where blood is purified.

---

1. French physiologist René Quinton (1867–1925) is best known for his Celtic sea water plasma clinics throughout France and his monumental study of the healing properties of sea water. He belongs to the elite group of Claude Bernard, Bogomoletz, and Walter B. Cannon, who advanced that the wisdom of the body consists in maintaining the integrity of its internal fluids.

Max Retschlag, a German alchemist who died in the 1930s, sums it up this way:

Our knowledge on the constitution of the human body, the structure of the cells and that of the smallest living entities leads us to rightfully believe that a certain remedy can be found, made up of a latent and concentrated energy, that will act as a universal remedy for all illnesses. Since the vital energy is a non-electromotive force, this specific remedy must be composed of matter capable of liberating a concentrated electric charge, after that matter has dissolved in the body fluids, just as it occurs in galvanic batteries where certain salts whose dissolution produces a more or less constant current between the poles.

From the large number of allusions made by the classic hermetic masters, it would appear that it is those same salts that enter as base material in the preparation of the elixir of life.

According to the broadest meaning of these alchemists, salt is defined as anything that crystallizes. Quoting these ancient masters, "Salt is the very first being since all matter can be reduced to the saline form. It is the Word of God turned into matter."

In pure salt, created out of the divine solar fire, this matter of celestial origin unites to passive earth in order to yield a saline incarnation. Chemically or alchemically speaking, this salt is made up of a mercurial humidity and of a sulphurous fat, and these two essences, antagonistic yet complementary to one another, form the original trinity of life as: alkali, acid and salt. Salt remains forever true to its form. Its crystalline living soul constantly gives birth to the same configuration; only the location and the circumstances of its origin change. Alchemic medicine thus avoids any remedy acting only materially; that is, the mere physical action of a remedy on the organism. It much prefers to effect the cure "from above," i.e., by a subtle healing action obtained from the heavenly forces. Whatever the various realms that alchemical medicine covers, the preferred method of the magisters is through the use of pure cosmic energy, the power of light and of vibration.

Alexander von Bernus (1880- - 1972) gives another quote, this time from an anonymous author from the end of the eighteenth century, the hermetic work entitled *The Secret of Salt: The most noble Creation produced by the great Goodness of God in the entire Realm of Nature*: "The salt is derived from the ashes of a great power... and there are virtues hidden therein."

To say that salt is "the Word of God" is not simply an allegorical allusion. It is no coincidence that the amniotic fluid that bathes the human embryo is salty and grey like the ocean from which all life on this planet has issued forth. Nor is it a coincidence that the most healing salt today is a "total" salt, with over 70 trace minerals, obtainable only by sun-drying and not by kiln- or flash pan-drying as modern refined salt is. It is also remarkable that alchemists accept only drying by the sun, since only that process would sublimate all of the noble minerals of the cosmos into the sea salt such as calcium, sulfur, phosphorus, potassium, and magnesium and all of the trace elements as well: copper, bromine, tin, rubidium, manganese, iodine, boron, cobalt, lithium, valine, nickel, fluor, chromium, silver, zinc and gold included. These macro-nutrients and trace elements are totally removed when modern refined table salt is kiln-dried and flash-crystallized. The alchemist magisters of old knew the difference somehow and that is why they spelled out: "Total" salt, obtained by the drying action of the sun and obtained from the sea, not from mines.

In the alchemic Art, sulfur and mercury stand for the two antagonistic properties of matter that are found everywhere in the cosmos. In the trilogy of sulfur, mercury and salt, salt represents the means of uniting these two first principles. However, we must bear in mind that sulfur and mercury are not describing the chemical element known to us by that name but define only certain qualities and properties of it. The salt that results from the fusion of mercury and sulfur can be compared to that vital spiritual force that permits the union of body and soul, the true anima that enables all creatures to become or stay alive, like Dr. Carrel's chicken heart. Because that knowledge has been passed to us in the form of symbolic images, sulfur was represented by a king robed in red and mercury by a queen in a white gown. Salt, which unites them, was always shown as a priest celebrating their marriage.

The philosopher's stone, as described by **Paracelsus** (1493 - –1541), was to "present a dazzling red color, that of rubies, and be sparkling and heavy. It heals the human body of all weaknesses and restores its health." I have seen such a substance in the form of traditional salt on a Pacific island, red as rubies and sparkling. Outside of the fairly sophisticated Celtic salt farms, it stands as one of the last sea salts hand-harvested by natives on this planet. It is never sold but is valued on a par with gold and the foreign visitors who overlook the experiencing of this true elixir are missing both the culinary experience as well as the energetic boost that this sublime element brings. The brilliant color of the aboriginal salt is obtained by the admixing of a special clay that the natives carefully measure into the salt brine as it crystallizes under the blazing tropical sun. They firmly believe this salt to be the human body's panacea for maintaining health as well as the integrity of their race. It may just be folklore, but it has been faithfully preserved in the course of their island-hopping migration from the Orient.

A formula given by the Belgian alchemist **Van Helmont**, who worked in Vilvorde, and by **Arnauld de Villeneuve** describes the power of this salty philosopher's stone as: "Having the property to create the form and perfect it infinitely since the improved form will improve the next and so forth till infinity."

The similarity between the division of living cells to form an embryo and the work of transmutation performed by the philosopher's stone does not end there. The analogy to atomic fission and chain reaction comes to mind and here also we see the deep wisdom that explains the alchemists' reluctance to divulge the Secret to the uninitiated, the same caution that prompted **Dr. E. Orowan** to state:

> The majority of earth's population considers that science and technology pose a growing deadly danger to their life. They feel powerless, at the mercy of the scientific minority, as if they laid on an operating table at the hands of, not healers, but of irresponsible playboys urged by curiosity or—what is worse—by a desire for notoriety or promotion.

When the first atomic bomb was dropped on Nagasaki, the only true protection and the only substance that saved many (who were closer to the epicenter than others who died) was none other than salty miso, a fermentation of soy beans and sea salt having a definite property for replenishing human body fluids with salt's minerals. While this panacea might not have been what the magisters of the Dark Ages had in mind for saving the human race back then, their refusal to allow the disclosure of their hermetic science to anyone outside their secret lodge, including the likes of today's mad scientists, was very much on their mind. The revelation of certain atomic secrets to irresponsible scientists has definitely put humanity in the grave peril of total extinction.

Isaac Newton (1642 - -1727) was both an alchemist and a "magician." I use the latter term because he considered the universe as an enigma, a secret that can be understood only by the application of pure thought to interpret certain phenomena. Sir Newton also thought that the indications that led to the solution of these enigmas could be found in part in the energy of the sky and in the transmutation of the chemical elements of earth and ocean. Newton highly valued the occult traditions and maintained the secret code of the documents that have been transmitted without interruption since the first cryptic revelations of the Babylonians about 10,000 years ago. After Newton, the idea that knowledge of the Art implied danger was overlooked and the ten-millennium secrecy of alchemy was broken. When the Emerald Tablet concludes, "The operation of the sun is complete," its author seemed to know that the planets and the stars draw their energy from the transmutation of the elements. What Paracelsus calls "the operation of the sun" is the very basis of the atomic bomb's construction—Fission–Fusion–Fission—that threatens to destroy our world today. Wouldn't it have been better if the secret of the operation of the sun had remained in the hermetic knowledge? The legend that too often identified alchemy only with the pursuit of making gold is false. It appears that the true dedicated initiates had little or no interest in gold but found that iron was much more important because iron is the origin, the ever-balancing beam of the universe.

A German alchemist wrote: "Eisen tragt das Geheimnis des Magnetismus und das Geheimnis des Blutes." Translated: "Iron carries the mystery of magnetism and the mystery of the blood."

In 1616, in the "Noces Chymiques," the formula with the atomic weight or iron isotope was revealed:

$$A=1, \ L=12, \ C=3, \ H=8, \ I=9, \ M=13, \ I=9, \ A=1, \ total=5$$

Iron with salt, with the latter capable of dissolving the first, are the essential constituents of blood, hemoglobin, and thus of life. Both of these elements are found, as a single pair or in combination, in human blood. The combination of salt (sodium chloride) with all of the macro- and trace elements present in natural sea salt plus iron make up the entire magnetic cosmos.

In every corner of the globe there lived masters who retained fragments of the secret teachings and divulged them to non-initiates. Here and there, parcels of the Art were revealed to the non-immortals: Porcelain, gunpowder, acids and gases. Electricity was known and jealously guarded in secrecy by the Baghdad alchemists in the second century, and Chinese alchemists produced aluminum in that same century by a process that leaked out only recently. And Sir Newton wrote in 1676: "There are further secrets besides the transmutation of metals and only the great magisters are to understand these." No matter how improper or dangerous these leaks of part of the great Art were, we must now entertain the possibility that the new alchemy offers, to a cruel world where death roams for all and nuclear accidents lurk at every turn, the chance of recapturing the true source and harmony of life.

Alchemy's altruistic attitude is still an exemplary force. It can become a guide and lead all of humanity to hope again. The day will come when all people will arrive at the full knowledge of alchemy in its pure thought form. It will then no longer be a physical science but an ethic of living. Most likely before the end of this century humanity will have to take this giant step of transmutation predicted by **Teilhard de Chardin** when he speaks of the "Grand mutation of humanity toward salvation." The secret of "the flowers of the waves" has yet to be revealed to all of humanity since there is not one single grain of salt that is pure, sweet ocean water, sublimated by the sun, available to the modern populations of the U.S., China, or the USSR. With this threat to human sanity and peace, refined salt must not continue to spread aggression, madness, and loss of equilibrium. If alchemy is to be finally revealed, with a true grain of whole salt, it will have won its ultimate victory. The term *sweet* is used knowingly; in the plasma of Quinton, the bitterness of sea water has been naturally transmuted to the sweetness of saliva and other healthy and healing body fluids.

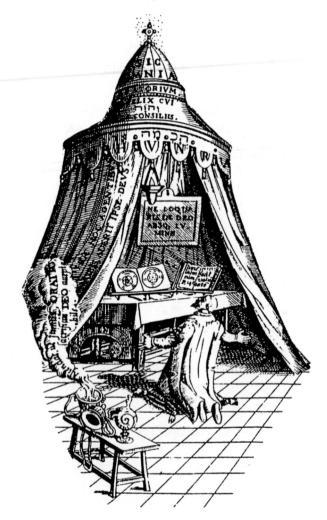

16

Beginnings

S HE wandered in an area where other tribe members had never dared venture before . . . but the familiar places had been picked bare and she was hungry and needed to gather some wild roots, meager subsistence for her man and child. Now next to the crashing waves and threatening surf her boldness wavered as she anxiously peered at a hollowed rock that the waves had filled earlier. Now the spin-drifts abated and the mist lifted. She saw the delicate white flower crystals that the salt brine had left behind.

Her heart quickened at the possibility that here was food; she bent close and her hand scooped some of the moist white crystals that floated on the now calm water. The pungent, salty and somewhat bitter taste stimulated and vitalized her. No longer hesitant, she gathered more of the white flowers and ran to the elders of the tribe.

The precious salt became an important complement to the tribe's food; the flower of the ocean also served as salve, medicine, and, in a very subtle way, caused some in the tribe to reflect and think. The tribe prospered, for they had found not only the condiment that made all roots and herbs taste and digest better, but the vital food that created human wisdom. Homo Sapiens was born.

Many centuries later, the human scientific mind began to dissect and analyze the dazzling white crystals. The rich minerals that bonded to that sea salt soon were stripped off and sold for profit as the first chemicals. The salt that remained no longer tasted sweet and pungent but caused insatiable thirst and anger. It no longer had the power to make people think, be wise and stay healthy . . . the mighty flower of the ocean had wilted and died.

Today, many of the same scientific leaders rightly accuse the modern refined salt of causing misery and sickness for humanity. Forbidding salt is not a solution. What is needed is the intuition that motivated that bold woman's gesture at the shore eons ago. Given a choice, her descendants today would rediscover the power of the flower and humankind would still be wise and smart. . . But then who is going to present scientists and statesmen with the true sea salt?

The search for better understanding of the flower of salt has not ended. As keepers of the ancient salt traditions, we are still seeking answers to the history and the mysteries of the divine essence. Part of the answer is in your hands but no one knows for how long. Celtic salt is hand-gathered by the salt farmers of Brittany and their technique and age-old craftsmanship is threatened by the giants of the drug and chemical empires. Sun-dried and unrefined, the flower is still moist, it has the might of the waves and the spin-drifts of the open seas, and the power to open the mind. Taste it and ponder its potential!

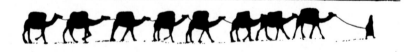

17

Most Often Asked Questions

Question: When shopping, I choose sea salt over plain salt since I believe it contains extra minerals. Is this a fact?

Answer: The term *sea salt* has lost its meaning. All the salt of this planet originally came from the sea, but more than three-quarters of all salt extracted today coming from (dry) fossil lakes and mines, this salt has not seen the sea for billions of years. What is worse, anything that is labelled "sea salt" today is always refined, having been subjected to total refining. Even health food store salt comes from those same refineries.

Whenever a natural food store or a food package boasts of having "sea salt," the truth is, every sea salt sold today has been refined by intense heat and recrystallized. All macrobiotic salts— and the miso, soy sauce and other products made from them —have also been desiccated and de-ionized. These processes have destroyed the antibiotic quality of these salts. Still-moist and unrefined natural Celtic sea salts, --sun- and wind-dried only-- harvested by the time-honored Celtic method, retain all of their natural qualities and taste.

Q: What makes natural Celtic sea salt superior to mine salt or to ancient seabed dry salts?

A: Biology research has proven that earth-bound salt lake and mine salts, even though they are unrefined and natural, are unbalanced in their trace elements. More important yet, these ancient sea beds have been stripped of many of their macro-nutrients, radio-vitality, micro-algae, oxygen, carbon dioxide and other vital gases. All these components are vital for the smooth functioning of our organism.

The biodynamic quality of sea water can best be demonstrated by a simple experiment. Living organisms such as brine shrimps—used commonly in labs to detect the presence of toxins—will not survive in refined or mine salt solutions. Pickles will also ferment poorly in the same salt. But the best test is your own body reactions; switching to Celtic sea salts for just a few days will most likely tell you clearly how your own body responds. No counselor or guru should presume to tell you which salt you should use. Natural hand harvested Celtic ocean salt alone helps to maintain life, neutralizes toxins and detrimental bacteria, and enhances all your organic functions.

Q: Isn't Celtic sea salt too yang (constrictive) compared to the "slightly refined" Lima, Muramoto and si-salts?

A: There are numerous yin elements in whole unrefined sea salt. Herman Aihara in his book *Acid and Alkaline* quotes from the book *Unique Principle* by Georges Ohsawa and restates that the following elements have shortwave radiation and thus are classified as yin: fluorine, nitrogen, phosphorus, sulfur, scandium, chromium, titanium, vanadium, calcium, potassium, nickel, manganese, iron, copper, cobalt, gallium, germanium, krypton, rhodium, ruthenium, molybdenum, antimony, cerium, lanthanum, praseodymium, terbium, europium, dysprosium, holmium, erbium, tungsten, osmium, bismuth.

All of these yin elements are destroyed whenever any artificial heat or boiling is applied. Oppositely, Celtic salt, having retained all of these yin and balancing elements, is effectively kinder to our biology and is, by far, more yin than these other salts.

Macro-nutrients in Celtic ocean salt make up 16% of the total solids, thus reducing the sodium level from 99% to 82%.

Regarding the terms *slightly refined* or *si-refined*, they are misleading since once the fossilizing or desiccating process has taken place, all precious and vital trace and macro-elements quickly vanish from the salt.

Q: Isn't sodium detrimental? Can we get too much sodium?

A: Sodium is the predominant cation of tissues, body fluids and blood plasma. Sodium is essential for digestive function, metabolism, nerve and muscular functions. However, the sodium in landlocked or refined salts hardens and has an altered molecular structure. This sodium will stubbornly remain in the body long after it has done its job, causing joints to swell (edema) and kidney problems. Unrefined Celtic salt has the opposite effect: its sodium drains out rapidly, keeping the kidneys at peak function, as well as promoting flexibility in the articulations.

Q: The presence of magnesium salts in Celtic appears to scare several health counselors. Can you elaborate on that point?

A: Far from being damaging, magnesium salts fulfill several important functions. First, sun-bright and magnetic, these salts eliminate fear and give courage to try new ways. They also brighten the spirit and promote independent thinking. By clearing the kidneys of stones and oxalate mud, magnesium salts, along with other precious trace elements, allow a thorough elimination of toxins while effectively flushing the body of excess sodium and calcium.

Sea water concentration of magnesium salts 0.33
Salt brine concentration of magnesium salts 16.85
Celtic salt concentration of magnesium salts 0.55
Muramoto salt concentration of magnesium salts 0.05
Si-salt concentration of magnesium salts 0.03
Morton, Leslie, & Diamond concentration of magnesium salts 0.01
(All above data obtained from analyses supplied by each manufacturer.)

Q: What are the esoteric aspects of Celtic sea salt?

A: This mineral is like unto the four elements—earth, air, fire and water. So universal, so necessary to life, it is the fifth element. Symbolically, salt is the extension of fire that issues from the earth mantle below the ocean floor. The movement of the tectonic plates creates newly formed or juvenile salt continuously, which explains why we instinctively choose and insist on obtaining sea salt in preference to land salt. The rites of passage always consist of placing a few moist crystals of sea salt on the tongue of the initiate or baptized. This ritual is still part of initiation ceremonies today. This step insures that the recipient will grow righteous, pure, and wise, by the powers inherited from God, their ancestors, as well as from salt, the essence of human enlightenment. These are granted to the ensuing generations by locking onto the akashic records. The akashic records are veiled memories of all events, thoughts and experiences that have inspired and guided humankind since the beginning of time. They are encoded in a fluidic ether that probes beyond the range of the five senses. That essence is encoded within the liquid mass of the planet. It is known in scientific terms as the pheromones, a hormone-like cell homing mechanism that is transmitted to human genes through air- and waterborne pathways. Before sinking into materialism, these human receptors were able to tune in, interpret, and heed these cosmic guides.

Insects, fishes, and mammals are still following their forebears' gene waves or pheromones but humans have lost this trait, possibly due to their alienation from nature's elements and support. In former times, our link with the watery depths of the planet was assured by our internal saline fluids and their affinity to sea water. Our daily replenishment with the total mineral spectrum from the planet's oceans stemmed from our most compelling instinct.

Q: Can this guidance technology of the human pheromones be verified scientifically?

A: Human pheromonal mechanism appears to be an encoding trapped within the moist crystal structure of natural sea salt, the guidepost that directs our genetic cells. The amino acids of the microflora (micro-algae) within the crystals are transported to the inner cells by our conductive internal saline solution. The nitrogen, mineralized by the salt's fixing agents, is absorbed by the aminic function that interacts with an algae-rich environment. This creates a new molecule, an amino acid that is intimately bonded to life by the following evolutionary characteristic: It appears sometimes as acid or as alkaline, depending on the circumstances. Regular molecules do not possess this ability to alter their pH—acid or alkaline—seemingly at will. This capability, called amphoteric quality,[1] is retained for as long as the salt crystal remains moist. The minute quantities of guidepost molecules, once regrouped in our body, constitute an action command post formed by a group of hormones, vitamins and diastases.

The urge to consume salt is far deeper than a preservation instinct. It is a powerful intuition that compels us to take salt extracted from the oceans of this planet and urges our instinct to seek and demand natural whole ocean salt in preference to the refined. That drive

---

1. Said of a substance that reacts with both acids and bases, acting as an acid in the presence of a base and as a base in the presence of an acid.

enables us to obtain all the minerals that are in the great oceanic cauldron. The sum total of human knowledge and character is transmitted to us by sea salt more than from any of the other four elements of the planet.

Q: Atomic radiation falls on much of the earth. How does this affect Celtic ocean salt?

A: The oceans receive much atomic fallout — the kind created by humans — actually more than land areas, but due to their salt and mineral contents, the oceans, and the natural salt produced from them, offer the strongest protection against man-made atomic radiation and fallout. (Salt mines and walls made of salt still constitute today the best possible containment for radioactive matter.) The power to stop or neutralize the effects of nuclear radiation on humans comes not just from the high percentage of sodium chloride in the salt but from the 16% other mineral compounds that strenghten immunity. Not the least the volatile organic iodine compounds. It is the combination of all these mineral elements in this symbiotic complex mix that enables Celtic ocean salt to cancel the effect of radiation on human and animal life.

But Celtic salt is also permeated with a beneficial radioactivity of its own, thought to emanate in the outer fluid region of the earth molten core, that is where 90 percent of the earth magnetic field originates. The salt's magnetism effectively opposes the man-made atomic fallout and is capable of cancelling the effects of the latter[1]. The force coming from the internal earth fire is further bolstered by the solar fire.

---

1. This was the experience of many residents of Nagasaki when the atom bomb fell. Those whose diet was salty: Miso, salt pickles and ume plums, suffered less from the effects of radiation.

Q: Gray salt does not dissolve completely. What is the effect of these undissolved elements on human biology?

A: Not every mineral in nature dissolves completely in water, yet their biological action on living organisms is positively effective. The undissolved matter in salt is biologically clean, made up of vital elements and composed mainly of metals, minerals, micro-algae, and plankton. The top surface of the oceans continuously destroys dirt; ocean air is totally free of atmospheric dust and pollutants; its salt, naturally extracted, is the only element that cleanses itself and also serves to protect and uphold our biological integrity.

The pure green-gray clay that lines the bottom of the salt ponds imparts a light gray color to the crystals. This is a pure, edible clay, an essential food that enhances the bio-energetic quality of the salt crystals and ionizes them as they form. Microbiology charts the various trace elements found only in unrefined crystal salt, and shows that, by their reactive properties, these micro nutrients positively affect the human organism.

In the final analysis, among all the salts of this planet, if we choose those that are sun-dried and harvested quickly by skilled hands from the remaining clean coastlines, we will enrich our body and spirit, and keep the spark in our life.

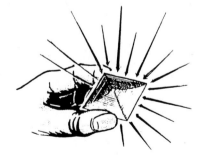

Bibliography

Books on the subject of salt abound. Rare are those works that study the sizable impact that natural ocean salt has on human biology. Some of the books and articles listed here supply small pieces of evidence that validate the ideas developed in the present volume. Others demonstrate how censorship insidiously works to destroy factual evidence. Of the two books bearing the same title (Colas, *Le Sel*, 1985; Stocker, *Le Sel*, 1949) and by the same academic press (Presses Universitaires de France), the more recent edition totally ignores the Brittany saltworks and willfully overlooks all natural salt production.

The media is self-serving and systematically eliminates embarrassing references. Since we aim to keep the true facts available to all, the honest works that expose or reveal, and truthfully cover, the complex issue of salt for humanity's sake have been marked by an asterisk (a double asterisk for an extremely strong recommendation). It may not make the establishment honest, but it will lessen the frustration in the seeker of factual information. Should any reader desire to obtain an out-of-print or currently suppressed work, the publisher will assist in locating it.

*Atkinson, Russell Frank. "Oceans of Life." *Nature and Health*, 1978. Melbourne, Australia.

Bergier, Jean-François. *Une Histoire du Sel*. Paris: Presses Universitaire de France, 1982.

Bertrand, Didier. *Le Magnésium et la Vie*. Paris: Presses Universitaire de France, 1967 [orig. publ. 1960].

Bloch, M. R. "The Social Influence of Salt." *Scientific American*, July 1963, 89–98.

Bonatti, Enrico. "The Origin of Metal Deposits in the Ocean Lithosphere." *Scientific American*, Feb. 1978, 54–61.

Boyer, Robert E. *Oceanography*. Northbrook, Ill.: Hubbard Press, 1974.

**Bressy, Pierre. *La Bio-Electronique et les Mystères de la Vie*, 2ᵉ édition. Paris: Le Courrier du Livre, 1979.

Britannica Books. *The Ocean: Mankind's Last Frontier*. New York: Bantam Books, 1978.

Bullard, Edward. "The Origin of the Oceans." *Scientific American*, Sept. 1969, 66–75.

Carey, George Washington and Inez Eudora Perry. *The Zodiac and the Salts of Salvation*. New York: Samuel Weiser, 1977 [orig. publ. 1932].

Choisel, Jean. *L'Avenir de Notre Évolution*. Paris: Courrier du Livre, 1964.

Clavel, Bernard. *Fleur de sel: Les Marais Salants de la Presqu'île guérandaise*. Paris: Chêne, 1977.

Colas, Alain. *Le Sel*. Paris: Presses Universitaires de France, 1985.

Denton, Derek. *The Hunger for Salt: An Anthropological, Physiological and Medical Analysis*. New York: Springer-Verlag, 1984.

*Dermeyer, Jean. *La Santé par l'eau de mer: Thalassothérapie*. Soissons: La Diffusion Nouvelle du Livre, 1972.

*Dickerson, Richard E. "Chemical Evolution and the Origin of Life." *Scientific American*, Sept. 1978, 70–87.

Dumas, Alexandre. *The Memoirs of a Physician*. Chicago and New York: Rand, McNally & Co., n.d.

*Edward, J. F. (M.D.). "Iodine in Prevention of Polio." *Manitoba Medical Review*, June 1954.

Encyclopédie Planète. *Trois Milliards d'Années de Vie*. Paris: Éditions Retz, n.d.

Engel, Leonard. *The Sea*. New York: Time-Life Books, 1961.

Eskew, Garnett Laidlaw. *Salt: The Fifth Element*. Chicago: J. G. Ferguson & Associates, 1948.

*Frieden, Earl. "The Chemical Elements of Life." *Scientific American*, July 1972, 52–60.

Hodge, D. C. "What's in the Sea." *Oceans Magazine*, Sept. 1982.

Hsü, Kenneth J. "When the Black Sea Was Drained." *Scientific American*, May 1978, 52–63.

Hsü, Kenneth J. "When the Mediterranean Dried Up." *Scientific American*, Dec. 1972, 27—36.

*Jannasch, Holger W and Carl O. Wirsen. "Microbial Life in the Deep Sea." *Scientific American*, June 1977, 42–52.

**Kervran, C. Louis. *Biological Transmutations*. Trans. Michel Abehsera. Magalia, Calif.: Happiness Press, 1988.

Kraske, Robert. *Crystals of Life: The Story of Salt.* Garden City, N.Y.: Doubleday & Co., 1968.

Krupp, E. C., ed. *In Search of Ancient Astronomies.* Garden City, N.Y.: Doubleday & Co., 1977.

*Kushi, Michio. "Dossier, Le Sel." *Le Compas,* Summer 1980. Vorey, France.

*Laragh, John H. (M.D.). "Giving Salt a Fair Shake." *Health.* Cornell Hypertensive Center, 1986.

*Lepierre, Charles. *A Indústria do Sal em Portugal.* Lisbon: Universidade Técnica de Lisboa, 1935.

Li, Choh Hao. "The ACTH Molecule." *Scientific American,* July 1963, 46-53.

*Liaisons Médicales Biologie Oligo-éléments. *Médecine Fonctionnelle des Oligo-éléments.* 16 avril 1978. Paris: Palais des Congrès.

*MacIntyre, Ferren. "The Top Millimeter of the Ocean." *Scientific American,* May 1974, 62-77.

MacIntrye, Ferren. "Why the Sea Is Salt." *Scientific American,* Nov. 1970, 104-115.

**Mahé, André. *Le Secret de Nos Origines.* Paris: La Colombe, 1962.

Meyer, Philippe. *L'Homme et le Sel: Rélexions sur l'Histoire Humaine et l'Évolution de la Médecine.* Paris: Fayard, 1982.

*Murray, Maynard. *Sea Energy Agriculture.* Augusta, Georgia: Sea Energy Agriculture, 1976.

Oort, Abraham H. "The Energy Cycle of the Earth." *Scientific American,* Sept. 1970, 54-63.

*Osterhaut, W. J. V. "Pure Salt is Poisonous." U.C. Berkeley Publication, Dec. 1905.

Penman, H. L. "The Water Cycle." *Scientific American,* Sept. 1970, 98-108.

*Poisbeau-Hémery, Jeanne. "Saliculture en Presqu'Ile Guérandaise."

**Quinton, René. *L'Eau de Mer Milieu Organique,* deuxième èdition. Paris: Masson et Cie, 1912.

Reinberg, Alain. *Le Sodium et la Vie.* Paris: Presses Universitaires de France, 1971 [orig. publ. 1964].

Revelle, Roger. "Man and the Sea." *Scientific American,* Sept. 1969, 3-13.

Revelle, Roger. "The Ocean." *Scientific American,* Sept. 1969, 54-65.

Rodale, J. I. *Magnesium: The Nutrient That Could Change Your Life.* New York: Harcourt Brace Jovanovich/Jove Publications, 1978 [orig. publ. 1968].

*Snively, William D. (M.D.). *The Sea of Life*. New York: David McKay, 1948.

**Société des Sciences Naturelles de l'Ouest de la France. *Marais Salants: Connaissance des Richesses Naturelles de la Loire-Atlantique*. Nantes: La Société des Sciences Naturelles de l'Ouest de la France, n.d.

Stephenson, Marilyn. "Warning on Salt Replacers and Potassium Chloride." *FDA Consumer*, HEW publication, 1979.

**Stocker, Jean. *Le Sel*. Paris: Presses Universitaires de France, 1949.

Wenke, Edward Jr. "The Physical Resources of the Ocean." *Scientific American*, Sept. 1969, 167–176.

Woodcock, A. H. "Salt and Rain." *Scientific American*, Oct. 1957, 2–7.

Wooster, Warren S. "The Ocean and Man." *Scientific American*, Sept. 1969, 218–234.

Index

Aberrant mental conditions 55
Aboriginal 28
Acid and alkaline 30
Acid-base 53
Acidic blood 31
Acidity 54
Acidosis 31
ACTH 51
Acute infection 56
Addicted 27
Addison's disease 54
ADH 50
Adrenal cortex 49-51
Adrenal glands 50
Adrenocorticalstropic hormones 51
Advertisements 24
Aerosolization 41, 44, 65
Aggression 77
Aging problems 31
Agro-fertilizers 11
Aihara, Herman 85
Akashic records 59
Albumen 54
Alchemists 63, 69
    Baghdad 76
    Chinese 76
Alchemy 7, 63, 64
    Arabic 70
    Chinese 64
Aldosterone 54
Algae 43
Algal 45, 48
Allergies 16, 54
Alumino-silicate 12
Aluminum 33
Amazons 51
Aminic-function 60
Amino acids 59
Ammonium 21
Amphoteric quality 60
Ancestors 5, 6, 9
Androgens 51
Androsterone 50
Anemic condition 27
Anger 79
Anhydrous 24
Animal protein 28, 29, 38
Antibiotics 27
Ancient alchemists 70
Antiseptic 61
Arthritis 56
Astral influence 63
Athrepsia 70

Atlantic 67
Atomic
    exposure 46
    fallout 47, 62
    fission 74
    radiation 46
    secrets 74
Attraction of opposites 51
Autoimmune disease 41

Babylonians 75
Bacilli 61
Bacteria 61
Bacterial diseases 54
Baghdad alchemists 76
Baking 33, 39
Baptism 59
Beer brewers 38
Benchmark 23
Bernus, Alexander von 72
Biochemical 29
Biochemistry 27
Biological deficiency 17
Biological functions 13, 15
Biological ineffectiveness 15
Biological necessity 13
Biological needs 12
Biological protection 62
Biological regulators 14
Biological requirements 15
Biologists 16
Biology 9, 13, 19, 48, 53
Biomedical research 55
Bitterns 16, 65, 66
Bleaching 33
Bleaching agents 24
Blocking 19
Blood 9
Blood of the Earth 70
Blood plasma 56
Body fluids 13, 55, 68
Boiled 15
Bone 56
    fracture 55
Boron 21, 68
Brain 56
Brain damage 30
Bran 39
Bread making 39
Brightness 22
Brine ponds 9
Briny salt pickles 64
Brittany 62, 67
Bromide 67
Bromine 72

Buffers 24
Burns 56
Butter-rich desserts 38

Cadmium 37
Cairn 7
Calcium 28, 30, 43, 55, 72
Cancer 54
Carbohydrate metabolism 56
Carbohydrates 28
Cardiac output 41
Carnivorous animals 29
Carnivorous humans 28
Carrel, Dr. Alexis 66
Cartilages 28
Catalysts 56
Catalyzer 19
Cattle 41
    feed 22
Caustic soda 12
Cell membranes
    "pumps" 30
Cell regeneration 30
Cellular energy 54
Cellular tissues 30
Celtic 7, 13, 14, 23
Celtic tradition 7
Celts 6, 7, 16, 65
Cereals 18
Cerebral hemorrhages 31
Chain reaction 74
Chardin, Teilhard de 76
Charred sea sponges 42
Chemical industry 68
Chemical iodine 43
Chemically-altered 27
Chemicals 11
Chew the bones 28
Chicken 41
China 64
Chinese pharmacopoeia 42
Chloride ions 35
Chlorine 35, 38
Chronic disease 30
City pollution 14
Civilized peoples 28
Clumping 14, 21
Co-action 30
Co-activity factor 19
Coastlines 47
Codex 24
Cold process 34
Coliform bacilli 61
Coloring 15

Commercial sodium chloride 24
Complex carbohydrates 28, 43
Condiment 78
Consciousness 58
Cooking 33
Copper 72
Cortex 50
Cortical hormones 49
Cortisol 50
Cortisone 50, 54
Cosmic ionization 61
Cosmic origin 7
Cosmos 63
Cows 27
Crabs 47
Cradle of life 7
Craving for salt 69
Craving for sweets 38
Cravings
  biochemical 29
  biological 29
Cretinism 41
Crude salt 37
Crystal structure 16, 32, 59
Cube 16
Cubic 22, 23
Cubic crystals 15, 16
Cultivated greens 27
Custom 8

Dark Ages 68, 74
Dead Sea 67
Deficiencies 19
Dehydration 16, 67, 68
Deity 7
Dementia 68
Depression 68
Desiccation 68
Dessicants 12
Dextrose 40
Diastases 60
Dietary supplementation 18
Dissolved gases 14
Distilled water 24, 31
Domesticated 27
Drinking the blood 28
Druids 7, 65

Earth and ocean 75
Eaux-mères 65
Ecologically 13
Edema 12
Egyptian pyramids 58
Electricity 76

Electro-magnetic 37
Electrolysis 43
Electrolytes 35, 55
Elixir of Immortality 64
Elixir of life 71
Emerald Tablet 69, 75
Emotional turmoil 56
Emulsify 38
Endemic goiter 41
Endocrinal system 47
Energetic boost 73
Energizing drink 33
England 9
Enigma 75
Enzymes 19, 21, 26, 56
Epilepsy 68
Estrogens 51
Eustatic ebb and flow 70
Evaporation 16
Excess consumption 37
Explosives 11

Fallout radiation 46
Farm animals 27
Fear of salt 16
Feces 55
Feminine reproductive
  system 51
Fermentation 38, 64
  natural 39
Filtration organs 51
First aid ointment 33
Fish 24, 43
Fission–Fusion–Fission 75
Flash crystallized 15, 65
Floods 58
Flower of salt 79
Fluor 72
Fluorine 21
Folklore 73
Folliculins 51
Folly 68
Foot rot 27
Free-running 34
Freeway crops 29
Fresh-killed animals 28
Frigidity 68
Fruits 18, 26, 27

Gabelles 67
Galvanic batteries 71
Gases 14
Gastric secretions 28
Gastric ulcers 31
Geiger counter 61
Genitalia 50

Geographic location 62
Germ 38, 39
Glandular 46
Glandular functions 50
Glandular tissues 40
Globe 14
Glucides 38, 54
Gnostic thought 70
Goiter 40, 41
Gold 72
Gold of the thousandth dawn 65
Gomashio 35
Gonads 49, 51
Goodness of God 72
Grain diet 38
Grains 26, 27
Grazing 26
Great Salt Lake 67
Greeks 42
Green leafy 37
Gunpowder 76

Hair 55
Harvest 23
Hay 27
Hayyan, Jabi ibn 66
Healing salt 72
Health food stores 22
Heart 28
Heat 24
Heaven and Earth 7
Heavy metals 37
Helmont, Van 74
Hemoglobin 49
Hemorrhage 56
Herbivorous animals 27, 29
High Middle Ages 67
Home process 37
Homo Sapiens 79
Hormones 54, 60, 68
Horses 27
Human blood 13, 30
Human body fluids 12
Human wisdom 79
Hunger for salt 59
Hydrochloric acid 38
Hyperactivity 41
Hyperplasia 41
Hypertension 31
Hypoplasia 43

Immortal spirit 58
Immortality 63
Immune response 16
Impotence 68

In vitro 61
Industrial revolution 11, 12
Infections 54
Inferior creations 69
Inland seas 10
Inorganic potassium iodide 40
Insatiable thirst 79
Instinct 9, 29
Integrity 16
Intelligence 7
Intestine 43
Iodine 21, 40, 41, 45, 67
Iodine supplementation 42
Iodized salt 40
Ion equilibrium 30
Ionic 55
Ionization 61
Ionize 44
Ionized 20, 21, 37
Ions 30
Iron 29, 55, 76
Isotonic concentration 60
Isotopes 55, 60
Ivanov, Mikhael 72

Jung, C. G. 70
Juvenile salt 65, 84

Kervran, Louis C. 63
Kidney cancer 54
Kidney failure 49
Kidney stones 56
Kidneys 36, 51-53, 68
Kiln 45
Kiln dried 15
Kiln-drying 24
Kosher salt 22

Laboratory 23
Land mines 59
Le Foch 61
Lead 37
"Lick" 9
Lifeblood of our planet 16
Lime 12
Lithium 21
Lobsters 47
Loeb, Jacques 23
Luster 22
Luteins 51

M.D.R. 40
Macro-minerals 24, 50
Macro-nutrients 18
Madness 77

Magisters 72, 76
Magnesium 24, 30, 50, 55, 67, 68, 72
Magnesium salts 12, 16, 27, 53, 56
Magnetic cosmos 76
Magnetismus 75
Making gold 75
Malabsorption 14
Mammary glands 41
Marine organisms 23
Marrow 28
Masculine regulators 50
Meat 27
Meat consumption 53
Meat eaters 28, 29
Meat tissues 27
Meat-based diet 28
Medical Congress 34
Mediterranean 67
Mending bones 60
Menopause 42
Menstrual irregularities 51
Mental disturbances 16
Mental equilibrium 67
Mercury 37, 73
Metabolic 19
Metabolic evidence 26
Metabolic functions 43
Metabolism 26, 54
Metabolized 18
Metal 33
Metallic ions 55
Micro doses 14
Micro-algae 7
Micro-dosages 56
Micro-doses 46
Micro-vegetation 48
Microchemistry 46
Microflora 60
Might of the waves 79
Mined salt 67
Mineral deficiency 15
Mineral sediment 33
Minerals 28
Miso 74
Miso makers 38
Modern civilization 28
Moisture 23, 24, 32
Molecules 20
Morality 7
Mother liquor 16, 23, 24, 34, 65, 69
Mother's waters 65
Muramoto salt 11, 85, 87
Mutation of humanity 76

Nagasaki 74
Nail 55
Natives 29
Natural experience 49
Natural unrefined sugar 15
Neolithic 9
Nephron breakdown 49
Nervous disorders 30
Neuralgia 31
Newton, Isaac 75
Nigari 34
Nitrate deposits 26
Nitrogenous intake 28
Nobel Prize 64
Non-immortals 76
Non-ionized form 17
Nutritive tissues 28

Obesity 41
Occult traditions 75
Ohsawa, Georges 85
Ohsawa, Lima 56
Oil 37
Oligo-elements 46
Oligotherapy 20
Operation of the sun 75
Organic iodine 47
Orient 66
Orowan, Dr. E. 74
Osmotic pressure 30, 60
Osteoporosis 56
Ovaries 42
Oversalted condition 54
Oxidation 16, 24
Oxydo-reduction potential 19
Oysters 47

Pacific Islands 29
Paludiers de Guerande 66
Panacea 73, 74
Paracelsus 73, 75
Parching 35
Particles 20
Parts per billion 21
Parts per million 20
Parts per trillion 21
Pathogenic bacteria 61
Pathological states 30
Pathology 42
Perspiration 68
Pesky flies 27
pH 19, 30
Pharmacy 64
Pheromonal manifestation 61
Pheromones 59
Philosopher's stone 73, 74

Phosphorus 21, 28, 43, 56, 72
Physical stability 14
Physical trauma 56
Physiology 9
Phyto-marine 61
Phytoplankton 49, 52
Pickle 38
Pigs 41
Pirenne, Henri 67
Pituitary gland 50
Plankton 59
Plasma of Quinton 69, 77
Plastics 11
Playboys 74
Poisonous 23
Polished rice 29
Pope Sylvester II 70
Porcelain 76
Pork 29
Potassium 29, 30, 55, 56, 72
Potassium iodide tablets 46
Potential 29, 30
Power of the flower 79
Pregnancy 42
Prehistoric 58
Prolongation of life 65
Protection 16
Protein-bound iodine 43
Proteins 28
Provider 50
Puberty 42

Queen 73
Quinton's Plasma 70

Radiation exposure 46
Radio-calcium 55, 60
Radio-iron 60
Radio-isotopes 60
Radio-manganese 60
Radio-phosphorus 60
Radio-magnesium 55
Radio-manganese 55
Radio-phosphorus 55
Radioactive 55
Radioactive iodine 46
Radioactive isotopes 55
Radioactive macro-elements 60
Radioactive trace elements 61
Radioactivity 61
Rains 58
Raw or cooked 26

Reabsorption of moisture 34
Reactivity 37
Realm of Nature 72
Recrystallized 22
Red ocher 29
Red Sea 67
Refineries 24
   multinational 37
Regenerates 9
Regulators 19
Retschlag, Max 71, 72
rH₂ 19
Rheumatism 31
Rickets 56
Rites of passage 58
Rock salt 5
Rocks
   granite 44
Roots and herbs 79
Rubidium 72
Runoffs 58

Saal 9
Sacred medicine 16
Safekeeping of minerals 32
Saline 69
Saliva 23, 28
Salt beds 9
Salt blocks 27
Salt box 17
Salt cellar 17
Salt flats
   concrete-lined 37
Salt starvation 17
Salt's integrity 15
Salt-poor proteins 28
Salt-starvation 27
Salting raw foods 27
Saltwort 47
Salve 78
Salzburg 9
Sauerkraut 65
Schmitt 61
Science and technology 74
Scientific minority 74
Sea algae 42
Sea vegetables 47
Seaweed 42, 47, 59
Secret of salt 72
Sensitive minerals 36
Sesame salt 35, 36
Severe burns 16
Sex organs 41
Sexual development 49
Sexual energy 52
Sexual mechanism 50

Sexuality 49
Shallow mine deposits 29
Sheep 27
Shipping lanes 62
Shock 56
Short-term 37
Shrimps 47
Silver 72
Skin diseases 54
Snack foods 27
Sodium 28, 30, 55
Sodium chloride 11, 23, 24, 26, 27, 29, 43, 52, 53, 65, 76
Sodium deficiency 26
Sodium iodide 40
Sour plums 64
Source of minerals 18
Soy sauce 36
Soybean paste 38
Spindrifts 41, 78, 79
Statesmen 79
Sterile 24
Stress 68
Strontium 21
Structure 22
Sublimation 63, 69
Sulfur 72, 73
Sun's rays 55
Supermarkets 22
Supplemented iodine 40
Surgical intervention 56
Switzerland 41
Symbiotic mix 62
Symbol of life 7
Symbolic images 73
Synergy 19

Tariffs 67
Technological intelligence 58
Testosterone 50
Thalassotherapy 34
The Art 64
Therapeutic 16
Therapeutic roles 12
Think logically 41
Thirst 36
Thyroid 43, 46
Thyroid gland 40, 42
Thyroid hormone 41
Thyroid malfunction 41
Thyroidal overdevelopment 40
Thyroxin 42, 43
Tin 44, 72

Tofu 34, 66
Top liquor 33
Total extinction 74
Toxic 18
Toxic effect 12
Toxicity 24
Toxicology 19
Trace elements 19, 21, 24, 29
Trace minerals 17, 18, 29, 51
Traditional gifts 8
Transmutable elements 27
Transmutation 7, 56, 63, 74-76
Tri-iodothyronine 43
Tribe members 78
Trilogy 73
Trilogy of substance 6
True anima 73

Unsalted raw diet 28
Unsalted raw foods 27
Urine 41, 47, 54
Uterus 42

Vacuum flash recrystallization 24
Vacuum-evaporated 15
Vacuum-processed 37
Vasopressin 50
Vegetable diet 36
Vegetable juices 36
Vegetables 18, 26, 27, 36, 39
Vegetal realm 26
Vegetarian animals 26
Vegetarianism 27
Villeneuve, Arnauld de 74

Violets 14
Virility 50
Vital essences 14
Vitamins 26
Volatile iodide 40
Vomiting 57

White flower crystals 78
Whole grains 38
Whole wheat flour 15
Wich 9
Wild 26, 27
Wild plants 26
Wild vegetation 26
Wisdom 58, 59
Word of God 71, 72

Yin-Yang 28-29
Yellow prussiate of soda 12

Zinc 72